AEROBIC DANCE:
A WAY TO FITNESS

Second Edition

Karen S. Mazzeo, M.Ed.
Judy Kisselle, M.Ed.
Bowling Green State University
Bowling Green, Ohio

MORTON PUBLISHING COMPANY
925 West Kenyon Avenue, Unit 4
Englewood, Colorado 80110

Printed in the United States of America

Edited by: Dianne J. Borneman
Illustrations by: Susan Strawn
Cover by: Dennis R. Walston, Certified Professional Photographer
Photography by: William E. Brown of Bowling Green, Ohio, and Dennis R. Walston of Canton, Ohio

Contents

Acknowledgements

Special appreciation is given to the following individuals who have shared their time and superb talents in this endeavor:

BGSU and BG community students
Robert E. Baird
Margaret E. Bobb
Richard W. Bowers, Ph.D.
William E. Brown
Roman G. Carek, Ph.D.
Mary L. Dieter
Mary Karen Dunlap
Sue Hager
Yonda Harrell
Jane E. Herrmann (deceased)
Carin Peirce Johnson
Timothy Kime
"Lerch"
Jeff Mack, Lake Erie Sports and Avia Aerobic 460 W Shoes
Gayle A. Marcin
Mary Beth Mazzeo
Michael Mazzeo
Lee A. Meserve, Ph.D.
Douglas N. Morton
Cynthia A. Oberfield
Bernard Rabin, Ed.D.
Jane Steinberg
Don Strait, Manager, Foot Locker—Franklin Park Mall, and Nike Air Aerobic Shoes
Student Recreation Center Staff of Bowling Green State University: Terry W. Parsons, Ph.D., Ron Zwierlein, Ph.D.
    Diana L. Muenger
Betty van der Smissen
Dennis R. Walston, C.P.P.
Laura Ware
Fran Weiss

A special thank you to the following for giving permission to use copyrighted materials:

The American College of Obstetricians and Gynecologists
Kris Berg, Ed.D.
Kenneth Cooper, M.D., M.P.H., and M. Evans, Publisher
The National Dairy Council
Michael Newton, M.D.
Frank M. Powell, Ph.D.
Jack H. Wilmore, Ph.D.
United Feature Syndicate and Charles Schultz

DEDICATION

To the very gifted individuals who shared their fitness skills and smiles to make this endeavor "visibly" magnificent! — "Butch," Mary Beth, Karen, Cindy, Gayle, Tim, "Lerch," Mike, Laura, Carin, Yonda, Fran, Mary, Moe, and Sue.
Thank You!

PREFACE

The fitness activity entitled "aerobic dance" has enjoyed unbelievable popularity and success in the past dozen years. It has survived the test of time from early critics as "merely a passing fad" to acquiring the distinction of having 18 million enthusiastic participants, and this number is skyrocketing daily!

With such a growing success story, it was understandable that a quality and informative course-oriented program describing basic principles and ideas was needed several years ago. **Aerobic Dance— A Way to Fitness** and **Aerobic Dance—Alternate Edition** were developed to provide that foundation. As with any body of health and fitness information, aerobic dance is dynamic. It is ever-growing and ever-changing and experiences not only new scientific findings constantly, but also new techniques—probably because of its intense popularity.

Aerobic Dance—A Way To Fitness, Second Edition provides you with just that. It updates the facts and blends the former two texts into one complete volume of information, requested by instructors as to format, and by students in terms of their needs. Since the text is designed primarily for the novice, explanations for developing a personalized program are given in a sequential but comprehensive learning order. Chapter 1 again establishes the basic definitions and principles, followed by Chapter 2 detailing the process for developing an individualized program.

Chapter 3 places a new and more detailed emphasis on body positioning (i.e., posture) for all movement so that this activity is not only **fun**, but also **safe fun** for you to enjoy as a life-time fitness activity.

Chapter 4 details the first portion of your workout hour—the warm-up. A basic routine is presented which will prepare the entire body, and all muscle and joint groups, for the intense workout ahead. Alternative options are also included to promote progression toward an advanced program.

Chapter 5 describes the ABCs of aerobic dance. It is a complete cataloging of step patterns, gestures, and sequence combinations—all listed alphabetically for easy learning and recall, and visually depicted in numerous photographs. The exercise movements have all been described and then photographed by a "mirrored" method. The student will easily understand that a movement described as using the **right** foot/arm/ or side of the body is **actually the left** foot/arm/side **of the model** (see Figure P-1). The student thus does

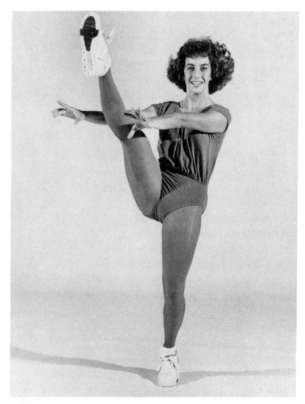

Figure P-1. With weight on your **right** foot, kick your **left** leg through both arms held parallel and extended forward.

not have to reverse the direction of what is pictured and what is performed! **You simply perform the movement on the same side of the body as you see it photographed and described.**

Note to Instructors:

When you teach as shown and described in this text, realize, of course, that when you say "weight on **right** foot," **you, the instructor**, are, as the model is, actually on your own **left** foot.

Chapter 6 completes the workout portion of the hour with cool-down stretching details and a sequential routine, followed with an optional strength-development program. Culminating the aerobic dance experience, then, is Chapter 7—the relaxation portion—which will complete the revitalizing process!

Chapter 8 encourages student independence by detailing the principles of choreography. Samples of several simple to complex choreographed dances are given to challenge all levels of skill and interest.

Chapters 9 and 10 on understanding body type, body composition, weight control, and a proper diet give balance to the text. To answer the many questions asked by individuals with special needs and concerns, Chapter 11 was created.

And, to determine whether established goals were met, Chapter 12 presents thoughts for evaluating your program.

The Appendix is extensive, providing numerous assessment techniques and monitoring charts to help you individualize your program. They are perforated and can easily be removed and turned in to an instructor.

1

AEROBIC DANCE:
A Definition

"I'm gonna live forever!" is a line in a recent popular tune. Some of us live our lives as if this were true—completely disregarding all personal self-discipline or pride in self and enjoying the easy life of overeating and underexercising. Our usual reasoning or excuse is lack of time. It usually takes a *crisis* situation to turn us around. But don't wait for a crisis. Set a priority—now—to develop a total fitness.

Physical conditioning through aerobic dance will assure you a happier, more vivacious, and abundant life. "We've moved beyond fantasy, to the reality that cardiovascular fitness can indeed reduce the risks of killer diseases and enhance the prospects for a longer, more energetic life."[1] And, some predictions are that by the end of this century the average American woman will live to age ninety, and the average American man to the mid-eighties.[2] With this projected long life ahead of us, let's make *sure* it will be a quality long life we're living by developing healthy life choices now.

Take a moment and fill out charts 1 and 2. Making a time commitment to yourself and profiling information about your self and your needs, wants, and goals is an important key way to begin your program.

Just What Is Aerobic Dance?

Most simply stated, the term "aerobic" means promoting the supply and use of oxygen. The body's demands for oxygen will increase when you engage in vigorous activity that produces specific beneficial changes in the body. Aerobic dance is an exciting and challenging fitness activity that combines exercise (exertion) and dance gesture and step patterns (rhythmical movement). It can be totally individualized so that you can move rhythmically to whatever beat (rhythm), whatever tempo (speed), and whatever form of movement you enjoy most—be it jogging, jumping jacks, or jazz moves! The three main criteria for aerobic dance movement that you *must include are:* **F.I.T.**

- The **frequency** of sessions per week;
- The **intensity** (how stressful the activity is); the intensity of movement must be maintained at a certain heart rate (beats per minute) in order for it to be truly labeled "aerobic dance"; and
- **Time duration** (spent per session).

The American College of Obstetricians and Gynecologists has developed and is actively promoting these safety guidelines, specific for aerobic dance: "To minimize the risk of overuse injuries during impact activities, it is recommended that the **intensity** should not exceed **75% of maximal heart rate**, the **duration** should not exceed **30 minutes**, and the **frequency** should not be greater than **every other day**."[3]

Precautions

If you have refrained from regular physical activity for a long time, have recently had surgery, are thirty-five or more years of age, are obese, or have specific limitations, you need a physician's approval to start this cardiorespiratory fitness program, as you would at the onset of any new vigorous work or leisure activity. A thorough medical examination is the recommended way to make sure that your current state of health and your physical capacity are adequate to safely engage in an aerobic dance program.

Aerobic Capacity Improvement— Your Main Objective

Aerobic dance significantly increases the oxygen supply to all body parts, including the heart and lungs, through continuous, rhythmic movement of large muscles and connective tissue. This type of movement conditions the body's oxygen transport system (the heart, lungs, blood, and blood vessels) to process the use of oxygen more efficiently. This efficiency in processing oxygen is called your "aerobic capacity" and is dependent on your ability to:

● Rapidly breathe large amounts of air
● Forcefully deliver large volumes of blood
● Effectively deliver oxygen to all parts of the body.

In short, your aerobic capacity depends upon efficient lungs, a powerful heart, and a good vascular system. Because it **reflects the conditions** of these vital organs, the **aerobic capacity** is the **best index (single measure) of overall physical fitness.**[4]

Measuring Aerobic Capacity

Pre-assessing your current status by having a thorough physical fitness exam will measure your heart's **response** to increasing amounts of exercise (work, stress) by measuring your ability to use oxygen.

Physical fitness can and should be measured in one of two ways at least every three years:

● A laboratory physical fitness test
● A field test administered by you and a friend

The Laboratory Physical Fitness Test

The "master key" to good health and exercising without fear is a properly conducted treadmill stress test to check out the precise condition of your heart.[5]

There's a difference between physical fitness and health, and the treadmill stress ECG helps to make that distinction.[6]

Before you are given a treadmill stress test, a thorough screening should occur. This consists of: (1) obtaining a brief history and physical exam during which the technician listens to your heart and lungs; (2) a check for the use of drugs that are known to affect the ECG (i.e., various heart and hypertensive medications); (3) a check for a history of congenital or acquired heart disorders; and (4) an evaluation of the resting ECG (twelve-lead). This can be recorded on chart 3. Participating in this screening and background check will help to determine your risk factors. A risk factor is a feature in a person's heredity, background, or present lifestyle that increases the likelihood of developing coronary heart disease.

Recommendations for Individuals at Higher Risk

An individual is classified as a higher risk candidate **if at least one** of the following factors is present:

1. Cigarette smoking
2. Elevated total cholesterol/high-density lipoprotein (HDL) cholesterol ratio (above 5.0 in males; 4.5 in females)
3. High blood pressure (greater than 145/95)
4. Abnormal resting ECG
5. Diabetes mellitus
6. Family history of coronary disease before, or by, age fifty.

★If **no symptoms are present**, an exercise test is not necessary below age thirty-five if guidelines mentioned earlier are followed.

★If **symptoms** of heart, lung, or metabolic disease **are present**, a maximum stress test is recommended for persons of any age, prior to the onset of a vigorous exercise program, and followed with tests every two years.[7]

Laboratory Testing: Sub-Maximal and Maximal Testing

Sub-maximal testing is accomplished by means of a physical fitness test (also called a stress test) on a moving treadmill. Electrocardiogram leads transmit and record electrical (heart) impulses that are read on a machine and recorded on a strip of paper. You are tested only to 150 beats per minute—not to exhaustion.

The ECG electrodes with leads are circular rubber discs that have wires attached to them. The discs are glued onto the chest and back at key locations so that various "pictures" of your heart—different angles and sides—can all be taken and recorded at once. Usually between seven and ten electrodes are applied, depending on the laboratory's procedures or on the individual's specific needs.

You will probably be asked to exercise (walk) at a pace of 3.3 miles per hour (90 meters per minute) on the moving treadmill. The grade will begin flat and will slowly increase in gradation, as if you were walking up a hill. Every minute the "hill" will become steeper and more difficult to climb. When your heart rate reaches 150 beats per minute, a record is made of the **time** it took for you to arrive at that reading. Then, through an indirect method of extrapolation (projection of maximum results through having tested many others the same way in the past), your fitness ability is estimated.

Basically, the **longer** it takes your heart rate to reach 150 beats per minute, the more fit you are; the **shorter** it takes, the less fit you are. Sub-maximal fitness testing is usually used for persons who have no outstanding limitations known to them, and who are interested in starting an aerobics program.

Maximal testing procedures are administered if an individual's need is more specific (i.e., for diagnostic or research purposes). Maximum testing **directly** reveals how much oxygen you use, because you are tested to exhaustion. The "exhaustion" point is when you start to get **markedly** fatigued. Some researchers feel that maximum laboratory testing is the **only** really conclusive type to use.

Field Tests of Fitness

You may not have immediate access to a laboratory and qualified physiologists to monitor the results recorded with the treadmill method. Therefore, included here are field tests that have been developed to help you assess your **own** physical fitness by determining your current aerobic capacity. This testing is easily conducted in an aerobic dance class setting.

The following information and tables 1-1 through 1-4 were developed from Dr. Kenneth H. Cooper's book, *The Aerobics Program for Total Well-Being.*[8] Cooper's Twelve-Minute Test and 1.5-Mile Test are two that you can administer by yourself or with the help

of a friend. Assess your cardiorespiratory endurance using one of these tests before you begin your aerobic dance program. **Re-assess** your cardiorespiratory efficiency **eight weeks later.** As aerobic dance becomes a lifetime activity for you, plan an ongoing assessment every two months. Compare your results with those from your first assessment. This will also help you set continual, life-long specific physical fitness goals.

Note: If you are over age thirty-five, it is strongly recommended that you start an aerobic dance program by first seeing your doctor, and then having a monitored **laboratory**-fitness test. And, individuals with **known** cardiovascular, pulmonary, or metabolic disease should have a maximum exercise test prior to beginning vigorous exercise at any age. These persons and persons with abnormal exercise tests should have a stress test annually.

Field Testing Guidelines and Procedures

1
Before undertaking either of these tests, it is strongly recommended that previously physically inactive people participate in one to two weeks of walking and/or slow jogging before testing themselves.

2
Wear loose clothing in which you can freely sweat and a sport shoe that conforms to the guidelines suggested in Chapter 2.

3
Determine first **which** field test you plan to take—running with TIME **or** DISTANCE as the stopping point.

- If TIME is the stopping point, take the twelve-minute test.
- If DISTANCE is the stopping point, take the 1.5-mile test.
- If you feel rather strongly that you are really out of shape, the twelve-minute test seems to be easier because you run for only this amount of time. (It may take an individual twenty minutes to complete 1.5 miles.)

4
Be sure that you have a stopwatch or a second-hand on your watch, or that you are close to a wall timer.

5
Immediately before performing the test, spend five to

ten minutes warming up the muscles (see Chapter 4).

6

Run or walk (or combination) as quickly as you can for a total of **twelve minutes**/or **1.5 miles**. This is an "all-out" test of endurance.

7

When you stop, identify precisely the distance covered.

8

Be sure to cool off (Chapter 6) by walking slowly for several minutes and performing cool-down stretching.

9

Interpret results for the **specified test** and **location** that you plan to use (tables 1-1, 1-2, 1-3, or 1-4).

10

Record your data on chart 4 in the Appendix, "Pre-Physical Fitness Testing and Appraisal Results" (A,B,C, or D), and then determine your fitness level. At the conclusion of your course, again assess fitness on chart 5, the "Post-Physical Fitness Testing and Appraisal Results" form.

Remember—for some beginners, the "good" performance level is very high. Do not be discouraged. You'll be pleased with your improvement as you participate in a **regular** aerobic dance program.

Understanding Fitness Test Results

"Good" and "high" on the laboratory testing and "good," "excellent," and "superior" categories on the field testing reflect that you are considered sufficiently **physically fit** to engage in a **continual** aerobics program.

If you place below "good" ("average," "fair," or "low") on laboratory tests, and "fair," "poor," or "very poor" on field tests, you are considered **physically unfit** and in need of a **conditioning** program.

Continual aerobics are performed non-stop for 20 to 30 minutes. **Conditioning aerobics** are intervals of exercise (the duration of one three-minute song, for example), followed by pulse-taking and recovery walking around for a one-minute interval. **Determining your fitness level, therefore, establishes for you the type of program in which to individually participate safely.**

Fitness for Life

Attaining a level of physical fitness entitled "good" or "high" (lab tests), or "good," "excellent," or "superior" (field tests) does **not** mean that you have achieved a finished product or goal. Instead, you have found a method of getting in shape that must be continued **for the rest of your life!** If you discontinue your program completely, all your aerobic gains will be lost in ten weeks.[13]

The need for personal fitness must, therefore, result in a complete change in lifestyle. You must prioritize and program exercise into your busy weekly schedule for the rest of your life. A "yo-yo" concept of a ten-week class now, and maybe one a year later, just doesn't maintain fitness and thus a healthy heart!

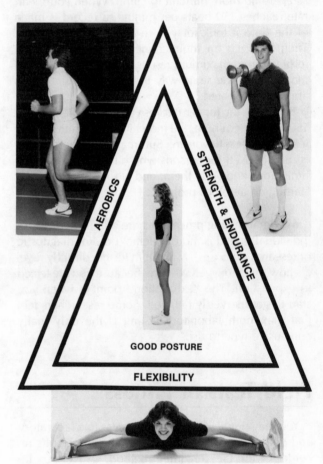

AEROBICS   STRENGTH & ENDURANCE

GOOD POSTURE

FLEXIBILITY

Figure 1-1.

The Total Physical Fitness Program

Total physical fitness is that positive state of well-being in which you have enough strength and energy

TABLE 1-1

Cooper's
12-Minute Walking/Running Test[9]
Distance (Miles) Covered in 12 Minutes

Use Appraisal A

Fitness Category		Age (years)					
		13-19	20-29	30-39	40-49	50-59	60+
I. Very Poor	(men)	<1.30	<1.22	<1.18	<1.14	<1.03	< .87
	(women)	<1.0	< .96	< .94	< .88	< .84	< .78
II. Poor	(men)	1.30-1.37	1.22-1.31	1.18-1.30	1.14-1.24	1.03-1.16	.87-102
	(women)	1.00-1.18	.96-1.11	.95-1.05	.88- .98	.84- .93	.78- .86
III. Fair	(men)	1.38-1.56	1.32-1.49	1.31-1.45	1.25-1.39	1.17-1.30	1.03-1.20
	(women)	1.19-1.29	1.12-1.22	1.06-1.18	.99-1.11	.94-1.05	.87- .98
IV. Good	(men)	1.57-1.72	1.50-1.64	1.46-1.56	1.40-1.53	1.31-1.44	1.21-1.32
	(women)	1.30-1.43	1.23-1.34	1.19-1.29	1.12-1.24	1.06-1.18	.99-1.09
V. Excellent	(men)	1.73-1.86	1.65-1.76	1.57-1.69	1.54-1.65	1.45-1.58	1.33-1.55
	(women)	1.44-1.51	1.35-1.45	1.30-1.39	1.25-1.34	1.19-1.30	1.10-1.18
VI. Superior	(men)	>1.87	>1.77	>1.70	>1.66	>1.59	>1.56
	(women)	>1.52	>1.46	>1.40	>1.35	>1.31	>1.19

*<Means "less than"; >"more than."

From THE AEROBICS PROGRAM FOR TOTAL WELL-BEING, by Kenneth H. Cooper, M.D., M.P.H. Copyright 1982 By Kenneth H. Cooper. Reprinted by permission of the publisher, M. Evans & Company, Inc., New York, N.Y. 10017.

TABLE 1-2
Cooper   12-Minute Run/Walk Test
Distance Expressed in ¼ laps for a 190 yd. track.[10]
Use Appraisal B.

Key: <=less than
     >=greater than

	Fitness Category	Sex	Age 13-19	Age 20-29	Age 30-39
"U N F I T"	I. Very Poor	Men	<12 Laps	<11¼ Laps	<10¾ Laps
		Women	<9¼ Laps	<8¾ Laps	<8¾ Laps
	II. Poor	Men	12-12½	11¼-12	10¾-12
		Women	9¼-10¾	8¾-10¼	8¾-9¾
	III. Fair	Men	12¾-14¼	12¼-13¾	>12-13¼
		Women	11-11¾	10½-11¼	>9¾-10¾
"F I T"	IV. Good	Men	14½-15¾	>13¾-15	13½-14¼
		Women	12-13¼	>11¼-12¼	11-11¾
	V. Excellent	Men	16-17¼	15¼-16¼	14½-15½
		Women	13½-14	12½-13¼	12-12¾
	VI. Superior	Men	>17½	>16½	>15¾
		Women	>14¼	>13½	>13

TABLE 1-3
Cooper 12-Minute Run/Walk Test
Laps and distances for a 126 yd. track[11] Use Appraisal C.

Laps	Distance	Women 13-19	20-29	30-39	Men 13-19	20-29	30-39
13	.93	Very Poor	Very Poor	Very Poor	Very Poor	Very Poor	Very Poor
13½	.96	Very Poor	Poor	Poor	Very Poor	Very Poor	Very Poor
14	1.00	Poor	Poor	Poor	Very Poor	Very Poor	Very Poor
14½	1:04	Poor	Poor	Poor	Very Poor	Very Poor	Very Poor
15	1.07	Poor	Poor	Fair	Very Poor	Very Poor	Very Poor
15½	1.11	Poor	Poor	Fair	Very Poor	Very Poor	Very Poor
16	1.15	Poor	Fair	Fair	Very Poor	Very Poor	Very Poor
16½	1.18	Poor	Fair	Fair	Very Poor	Very Poor	Poor
17	1.22	Fair	Fair	**Good**	Very Poor	Poor	Poor
17½	1.25	Fair	**Good**	Good	Very Poor	Poor	Poor
18	1.29	Fair	Good	Good	Very Poor	Poor	Poor
18½	1.32	**Good**	Good	Excellent	Poor	Fair	Fair
19	1.36	Good	Excellent	Excellent	Poor	Fair	Fair
19½	1.40	Good	Excellent	Excellent	Fair	Fair	Fair
20	1.43	Good	Excellent	Superior	Fair	Fair	Fair
20½	1.47	Excellent	Superior	Superior	Fair	Fair	**Good**
21	1.50	Excellent	Superior	Superior	Fair	**Good**	Good
21½	1.54	Superior	Superior	Superior	Fair	Good	Good
22	1.58	Superior	Superior	Superior	**Good**	Good	Excellent
22½	1.61	Superior	Superior	Superior	Good	Good	Excellent
23	1.65	Superior	Superior	Superior	Good	Excellent	Excellent
23½	1.68	Superior	Superior	Superior	Good	Excellent	Excellent
24	1.72	Superior	Superior	Superior	Good	Excellent	Superior
24½	1.75	Superior	Superior	Superior	Excellent	Excellent	Superior
25	1.79	Superior	Superior	Superior	Excellent	Superior	Superior
25½	1.83	Superior	Superior	Superior	Excellent	Superior	Superior
26	1.86	Superior	Superior	Superior	Excellent	Superior	Superior
26½	1.90	Superior	Superior	Superior	Superior	Superior	Superior

TABLE 1-4
Coopers 12-Minute Run/Walk Test
Time (Minutes)[12]
Use Appraisal D.

Key: <=less than
>=greater than

		Age	Age	Age
Fitness Category	**Sex**	**13-19**	**20-29**	**30-39**
I. Very Poor	Men	**>15:31	>16:01	>16:31
	Women	>18:31	>19:01	>19:31
II. Poor	Men	12:11-15:30	14:01-16:00	14:44-16:30
	Women	18:30-16:55	19:00-18:31	19:30-19:01
III. Fair	Men	10:49-12:10	12:01-14:00	12:31-14:45
	Women	16:54-14:31	18:30-	19:00-16:31
IV. Good	Men	9:41-10:48	10:46-12:00	11:01-12:30
	Women	14:30-12:30	15:54-13:31	16:30-14:31
V. Excellent	Men	8:37-9:40	9:45-10:45	10:00-11:00
	Women	12:29-11:50	13:30-12:30	14:30-13:00
VI. Superior	Men	<8:37	<9:45	<10:00
	Women	<11:50	<12:30	<13:00

From **THE AEROBICS PROGRAM FOR TOTAL WELL-BEING**, by Kenneth H. Cooper, M.D., M.P.H., Copyright 1982 by Kenneth H. Cooper. Reprinted by permission of the publisher, M. Evans and Company, Inc., New York, N.Y. 10017

to participate in a full active lifestyle of your own choice.

A **total** fitness program consists of three basic parts and can be visualized by the fitness triangle (figure 1-1):

1

Aerobic (cardiovascular and respiratory) fitness (already explained).

2

Flexibility (ability to bend and stretch).

3

Muscular strength and muscular endurance training (thickening muscle fiber mass to enable individuals to endure a heavier work load).

More specifically, **flexibility** is the range of motion of a certain joint and its corresponding muscle groups. The greater the range of movement, the more the muscles, tendons, and ligaments can flex or bend. Muscles are arranged in pairs. One muscle's ability to shorten or contract is directly related to the opposing muscle's length or stretch. Flexibility is maintained or increased by movement patterns that slowly and progressively stretch the muscle beyond its relaxed length.

Muscular strength is the ability of a muscle to exert a force against a resistance. Strength activities increase the amount of force that muscles can exert or the

amount of work that muscles can perform. Activities such as weight training can develop powerful muscles. Still, they do not provide a vigorous increased usage of **oxygen** to condition the **heart** to function more efficiently, as does aerobic activity.

Muscular endurance is the ability of muscles to work strenuously for progressively longer periods of time without fatigue. It is the capacity of a muscle to exert a force **repeatedly** or to **hold** a static (still) contraction over a period of time.

A total, well-rounded weekly fitness program should consist of regular participation in **all three components**. However, since the sign of genuine fitness is the condition of your heart, your blood vessels, and your lungs, **aerobic fitness** is the most important component.[14] By engaging in aerobic dancing (or any aerobic activity), your heart gradually strengthens and develops a greater capacity to pump more oxygenated blood to the body with fewer contractions (exercised hearts are stronger and slower).

Highly trained and conditioned endurance athletes have **resting** heart rates as low as 30 to 32 beats per minute, an unbelievably low rate! What actually happens is that with regular, stimulating exercise, the heart becomes a more efficient pump. It pumps more blood with each stroke, and with a more efficient stroke volume, your heart can function with less effort. By getting your heart into condition, you may be practicing preventive medicine. You may be lessening the danger of a coronary heart attack, five, ten, fifteen, twenty years from now. And if you do have one, your chances of surviving are far greater with a heart, and lungs, and blood vessels which are in good condition.[15]

It is thought-provoking to realize that you can still exist without big bulging muscles, or without the perfect figure, or with a head cold—but that you can't exist very long without a good heart and lungs. Unfortunately, more than 40 percent of all people who have their first heart attack do not receive a second chance to change their habits, or develop an aerobic program—they die.[16] And over one-half of all American deaths last year were due to heart-related diseases.[17] If only we could establish a living pattern priority **early** in life to correct this overwhelming statistic.

Strengthening the Heart: Progressive Overload Principle

Aerobic dance, like any aerobic activity, conditions the heart to **strengthen it** through a principle called "progressive overload." Not only will the heart pump more blood each beat, it will have longer rests between each beat, therefore lowering the pulse rate. Aerobic dance "overloads" the heart by causing it to beat faster during the vigorous workout, making a temporary high demand on the cardiorespiratory system. As you become more fit, the heart eventually adjusts to this demand and soon is able to do the same amount of work with less effort.

Aerobic Versus Anaerobic Dance

Very simply stated, all **aerobic** activity has several essential criteria that must be present in order for the exercise to be labeled "aerobic." Since "aerobic" means "with oxygen," the movement that you do must:

1

Use the **large** muscles of the body (like your arms and legs).

2

Be **rhythmic** ("one-two-one-two").

3

Be **continuous** for a twenty-to-thirty-minute **duration of time** (actually, fifteen to sixty minutes, according to **intensity**—how stressful the activity is).

4

Be practiced for a **frequency minimum of three sessions per week.**

- Four days a week or "every other day" is good.
- Some key researchers state five days is a maximum for fitness goals. Beyond this injuries are ten times more likely to occur to the musculo-skeletal system from overuse. Give your body at least two days of rest.

5

And, in order to receive the cardiovascular fitness benefits, called the "training effect," the **heart rate must be maintained in a specific "training zone"— the individualized safe pace** at which to aerobically work or exercise. This reflects your **intensity** and is scientifically explained as a percentage of your maximum heart rate or maximum oxygen uptake. Intensity is discussed in more detail throughout the remainder of this chapter.

Any activity that fits these aforementioned five criteria would be considered **aerobic.**

Anaerobic activity, then, is basically activity that is "stop and start," or one in which the heart is not kept at a constant steady pace for fifteen to sixty minutes (or more in the case of marathons). Thus, "anaerobic" describes an activity that requires an all-out effort of short duration and that does not utilize oxygen to produce energy. This type of exercise quickly uses up more oxygen than the body can take in while engaging in the exercise, causing an oxygen debt. This, in turn, causes lactic acids (waste products) to accumulate in the muscles, which leads to exhaustion.

What Is Individual Intensity?

As briefly mentioned earlier, intensity means how stressful the activity is and is explained (or "measured," or "monitored") as a percentage of your maximum heart rate. A specific individualized intensity is maintained by each participant during each session of aerobic dance. The intensity at which each individual works is reflected or described as the estimated **safe** range in which to exercise. This is determined by your **age** (unless you have heart problems or other limitations), your **lifestyle**, and the variable of your **resting heart rate** also considered. Details for persons with limitations are given in Chapter 11.

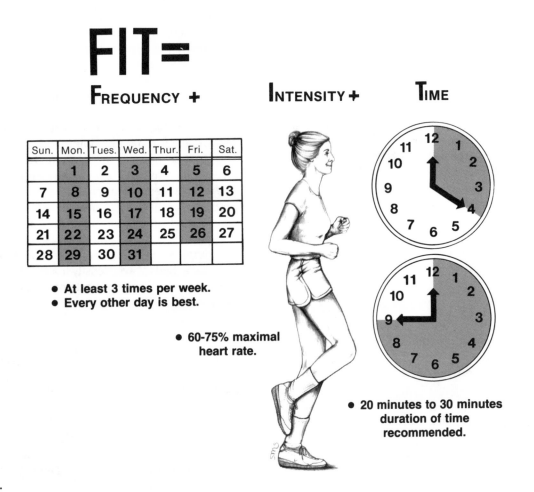

FIT=

FREQUENCY +   **INTENSITY +**   **TIME**

Sun.	Mon.	Tues.	Wed.	Thur.	Fri.	Sat.
	1	2	3	4	5	6
7	8	9	10	11	12	13
14	15	16	17	18	19	20
21	22	23	24	25	26	27
28	29	30	31			

- At least 3 times per week.
- Every other day is best.

- 60-75% maximal heart rate.

- 20 minutes to 30 minutes duration of time recommended.

Figure 1-2.

Training Zone Heart Rate

This is the individualized safe exercise zone in which to aerobically work, i.e., exercise—be it aerobic dance or any other aerobic activity. In order to receive the cardiorespiratory fitness benefits, called the "training effect," of any aerobic activity, the heart rate must be maintained in a specific training zone.

It's A Pulse-Monitored Activity

To insure that each individual learns how to **steadily pace** oneself for a **duration** (endurance) activity, learning how, when, and why to monitor the heart rate is one of the initial skills taught in aerobics programs. Once the pulse is taken, each individual records, on paper, what has been monitored.

How To Monitor Your Heart Rate

The pulse equals heartbeats per minute and can be felt and counted in one of six pulsation points. Select at which area you can best obtain a pulse, using your index and second fingers. The two places most often used for pulse counting are on the neck, near the carotid artery, and on the wrist, near the radial artery.

1

The carotid artery runs up the neck and is usually easy to find. Place your index and middle fingers **below the point of your jawbone** and slide downward an inch or so, pressing lightly. When you use the carotid artery pulse-monitoring method, make sure that you apply light pressure, as excessive pressure may cause the heart rate to slow down by reflex action.

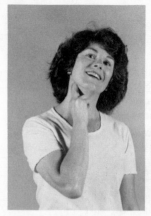

Figure 1-3.
Taking the carotid pulse.

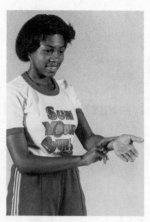

Figure 1-4.
Taking the radial pulse.

2

The radial artery runs up the wrist on the **thumb side**. Place your index and middle fingers just below the base of your thumb. Press lightly. Now count the number of pulsations, or beats, in one of three ways. For each:

- Six seconds and multiply by 10 (i.e., add a zero to pulse felt).
- Ten seconds and multiply by 6.
- Fifteen seconds and multiply by 4.

Once the pulse is taken, each individual records, on paper, what has been monitored. **The total is the number of heartbeats per minute.** To count correctly, make sure that you count each beat you feel.

Your heart rate will increase after vigorous aerobic activity and should return to normal within a short period of time after resting. As a rule, the faster it slows down (i.e., recovers from exercise), the more physically fit you are.

Your Goal: To Achieve the Training Effect

By "overloading" the heart with vigorous aerobic dancing, your aerobic capacity is increased and a desirable **training effect** can be achieved. The training effect, or total beneficial changes that usually occur are:

- Stronger heart sending more oxygenated blood to all tissues of the body.
- More blood cells produced.

- Slower resting heart rate.
- Expansion of blood vessels.
- Improvement of muscle tone.
- A lowering of blood pressure for some through improved circulation.
- Stronger respiratory muscles.
- Regulates the release of adrenalin.
- Increased lung capacity.
- A more regular elimination of solid wastes.
- Lower levels of fat found in blood.[19]
- Strengthens muscles and skeleton to protect them from injury in later life; by increasing bone density, it helps prevent osteoporosis.[20]
- Increased sensitivity to insulin and lowered blood sugar levels in mild, adult-onset diabetes.[21]
- Improves the way cholesterol is handled by the body, by increasing the proportion of blood cholesterol attached to high-density lipoprotein—a carrier molecule that keeps cholesterol from damaging artery walls.[22]

Benefits of Aerobic Dance

Achieving the training effect, and therefore numerous beneficial physiological changes, will carry over into all of your daily living. A high fitness level will give you more energy to live life to its fullest. Once on the path toward fitness, you will be able to handle stressful situations, daily tasks, and emergencies better than before. Your mental capabilities—including better concentration—will also improve. You will have established a self-discipline toward keeping unwanted fat pounds away—that is, if your eating habits have been improved! And, as you incorporate correct posture through correct (efficient) aerobic dance movement, you will be working toward eliminating sagging abdominal muscles and toward strengthening weak back muscles associated with lower back pain. This new efficiency will then, very naturally, carry over into **all** of your daily work and leisure activities, providing you with a more comfortable, quality day.

People who engage in a **regular** program of aerobic dance will tell you from their own experience that they look and feel much better about themselves! As you begin achieving your fitness goals, the feeling of pride in yourself will surface and do wonders to boost your self-confidence. And, as you feel more positive about **yourself**, you will also develop a more positive attitude **toward others**. Just think what a fantastic impact this one particular fitness benefit can have on your life!

All of the above are incentives for starting and continuing an aerobic dance program. As you can see, the benefits are numerous!

Aerobic Alternatives

Other aerobic activities with which you can supplement your **aerobic dance** program include:

- Cross-country skiing.
- Cycling (includes stationary cycling).
- Jogging/Running.
- Jumping Rope.
- Rowing.
- Swimming.
- Walking (moderate to fast pace-walk).

Like aerobic dance, these vigorous, continuous, and rhythmic activities are excellent because they condition the cardiorespiratory system and increase its efficiency by demanding large amounts of oxygen over an extended period of time. The more you participate in aerobic dancing or other aerobic activities, the better your heart adapts to stress (by regulating the release of adrenalin) and works with the lungs to pump more oxygen to the muscles and body tissues quickly. This explains why cardiorespiratory (heart, lungs, vessels) efficiency is the most important component of physical fitness.

The value of time
The virtue of patience
The success of perseverance
The influence of example
The improvement of talent
The joy of creativity!
. . . I reflect upon each,
while I discipline my flesh.
I realize
There is nothing more difficult,
than working against the flesh . . .
If I am successful,
it establishes a permanent
***Discipline**, a confidence,*
that allows me to do well
in everything else I try.

2

DEVELOPING YOUR OWN AEROBIC DANCE PROGRAM

"The constant movement of both arms and legs typical of most aerobic dance exercise programs provides a workout that can reach extremely high levels of intensity. Aerobic dance exercise is especially popular . . . because it includes aesthetic components lacking in other aerobic activities. Popular music enhances group dynamics and appears to mask the discomfort of strenuous training. The typical indoor environment also provides security and comfort for many . . ."[1]

This statement was made in a publication just released by a body of nationally acclaimed medical professionals. The medical profession is beginning to recognize the overwhelming popularity of aerobic dance and is establishing safety guidelines. These guidelines are long overdue for an activity that is proving to be the number one fitness activity choice of a skyrocketing number of Americans.

No wonder there is such a growing interest in **aerobic** dance. You have fun while you gain physiological **and** psychological benefits. You achieve a good feeling about yourself and develop a more positive self-image. Students of aerobic dance have so much fun that they sometimes forget they are actually exercising and participating in one of the most effective physical fitness programs available today. Also, aerobic dancing has the necessary elements to prevent exercise from becoming boring and tedious.

The Four-Segment Aerobic Dance Program

There are four essential aspects of a good aerobic dance program:

- A warm-up.
- Aerobic dance gestures and step patterns.
- A cool-down.
- Relaxation.

1 Warm-Up

Execute the warm-up stretching exercises with efficient posture for at least five, preferably ten minutes, in the order in which they are presented. As you warm up, you make all parts of your body more supple (Chapter 4).

2 Aerobic Dance Gesture and Step Patterns

Again, using efficient posture, start with a letter of the alphabet and perform the exercises several times until you know each well. As you confidently execute one basic exercise without hesitation or stopping, begin learning the next. Try a new exercise from the index list of possibilities only **after** you have mastered one.

Learn at your own pace. Learning in the order in which the exercises appear in the book is recommended **for easier recall**. This is, of course, strictly optional because understanding each gesture and step pattern does not require any prior skill—they are all uniquely different moves—one from the next.

The best learning progression for understanding a certain movement is dissecting it as follows:

- Perform first the step patterns to every other beat of the music (i.e., slow motion).
- Hasten the pace and move to every beat of the music.

- Add high-intensity and impact movement and perfect your body position with efficient, tight, excellent form.
- Add the arm gestures suggested.
- Create a variety of arm gestures to the movement.

Once you have mastered the indexed possibilities, it's time to place them into planned routines or dances, choreographed by an instructor or by you.

Keep dancing and keep moving in order to reach and remain in your training zone and therefore work toward experiencing and obtaining the training effect. "Overload" your heart so that cardiorespiratory fitness becomes a reality. Start with several minutes (perhaps one song) and keep adding as much time as you comfortably can (one several-minute song at a time) until you've engaged in at least twenty minutes of aerobic dancing. Working constantly in (approximately) three-minute **intervals**, with heart rate monitoring in between, will allow the new **unconditioned** dancer a safe way to begin exercising.

If aerobic dance is new to you, **but** you begin at a **high** level of fitness (pretest out to be in "good" or better condition on a fitness test), your program can be of a **continual**, high-intensity nature. Perform a minimum amount of heart rate monitoring. If you are in a conditioning course where the group works in intervals and/or frequently monitors the dancing heart rate, **you** engage instead in a high-intensity activity like jogging, jumping rope, reviewing what you've learned, or improvising movement that you enjoy (see Chapter 8 for ideas). This procedure individualizes the program hour so that everyone is working safely and toward the goals they've set for themselves. No one is working above or below their own safe level.

3 Cool-Down

Choose an activity and stretching exercises that slow down large muscle activity (Chapter 6). Begin by slow dancing or walking for a minute or two, followed by **sitting** and then **lying** down while performing stretching exercises. If you complete a session by learning new basic movements or a new choreographed dance routine in which you just "walk" through it, you can count this activity as part of your cool-down. A **minimum** of **five minutes** is required for cool-down. Heart rate should be below 120 when you finish.

Note: If you wish to perform strength training exercises, **now** is the time in your program hour to do so.

4 Relaxation

The Voluntary Conscious Relaxation Technique given in Chapter 7 totally uses your powers of control through your **imagination**—your **mind** seeks out and recognizes tension in a four-phase process. This brings a refreshing conclusion to a physically challenging aerobic dance session. Be sure to give yourself these five or ten minutes (or more) to complete the whole energizing process of an aerobic hour. This final phase has become a favorite of each and every student who has experienced it.[2]

Remember To Make It Continually Aerobic

You will find as you progress with your program that you will increase:

1
The **frequency**—from the minimum of three days to a maximum of five days per week.

2
The **intensity**—gradually moving from the lower end of your training zone up to the top of your training zone by rhythmically and continuously using your large muscle groups in an increasingly more tense and firm fashion.

3
The **time duration**—lengthening the amount of time for each aerobic segment of your workout; i.e., from three-minute intervals, to thirty minutes of non-stop dancing.

Remember: Dancing at a high level of exertion for at least twenty minutes on a regular basis of at least three times a week is the key to an optimal level of fitness!

Gradual, Sensible— Don't Overdo It!

It takes a planned self-discipline to become and stay physically fit, but the dividends of wellness and vitality are well worth it.

Progress gradually and sensibly in your sessions. Remember to warm up and cool down and to progress from easy to hard—both in the stretches and in the aerobic combinations. Learn to read your body signs. You're going to perspire and you're going to tire **a little**, but keep performing. However, you do not need to perform to the point of exhaustion. Know that with an effective aerobic dance program you may encounter some initial, slight, temporary discomfort, so be sensible about pacing yourself. For example, after engaging in several aerobic dance movements or a complete dance routine, you may be short of breath, but this should subside within minutes after the activity. If it doesn't subside, you've worked too hard. If you are unsure about a particular discomfort or pain, ask a reliable person (such as your doctor) before you continue with the activity.

Definite Signs of Overexertion

Remember—while monitoring your pulse helps you determine how hard to exercise your body, you also need to be aware of your own bodily signs. Signs of overexertion are:

- Severe breathlessness.
- Poor heart rate response (continually monitoring too high a dancing heart rate that does not significantly drop after one minute recovery reading or final recovery rate not below 120 beats per minute after five minutes of cool-down).
- Undue fatigue during exercise and inability to recover from a workout later in the day.
- Inability to sleep at night.
- Persistent severe muscle soreness. (The type of muscle soreness to guard against is not the immediate type, but that which becomes apparent after twenty-four to forty-eight hours.[3] Refer to Chapter 11 for details.)
- Nausea, feeling faint, dizziness.
- Tightness or pains in the chest.

These symptoms do not mean that you should not exercise; rather, they suggest performing a reduced level of activity until you develop the capacity to handle more intense workouts. It is important to embark on an exercise program cautiously and to **increase gradually** the frequency, the intensity, and/or the time duration of your program.

If you have any of these symptoms, ease down to a slow walk, sit down with your head between your knees, or lie down on your back and elevate your feet. This will help the blood move to your head more easily and carry the needed oxygen to your brain. If any of these symptoms last longer than a brief period of time, contact your doctor.

Note: Seek medical advice immediately and before the next exercise session if any of these symptoms occur:

1 *Abnormal heart action*

- Pulse becoming irregular.
- Fluttering, jumping, or palpitations in chest or throat.
- Sudden burst of rapid heartbeats.
- Sudden, very slow pulse when a moment before it had been on target (immediate or delayed).

2 *Pain or pressure in the center of the chest or the arm or throat precipitated by exercise or following exercise (immediate or delayed).*

3 *Dizziness, light-headedness, sudden incoordination, confusion, cold sweat, glassy stare, pallor, blueness, or fainting (immediate).*

Do not try to cool down. Stop exercise and lie down with your feet elevated, or put your head down between your legs until the symptoms pass.[4] Information for various problems that frequent this activity are discussed in Chapter 11.

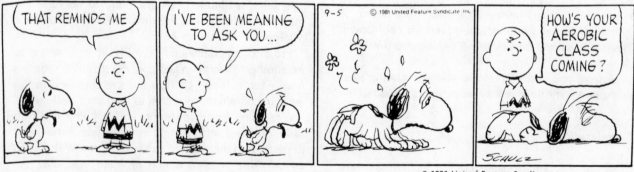

© 1981 United Feature Syndicate, Inc.

Self-Discipline: A Choice

It takes hard work to achieve physical fitness. There are no shortcuts or easy ways. Once achieved, you must keep working to maintain fitness for life. **Maintaining** fitness is a lot easier than initially **achieving** it. The less physically fit you are, the longer it will take to achieve fitness. You will need to count your progress in months as well as days. Fitness requires self-discipline and choices. **You** are in control—no one or nothing else can do it for you!

The Key: Enjoyment and Regularity

The key to maintaining a fitness program is to choose an aerobic activity that you truly enjoy and in which you can participate with enthusiasm and on a regular basis **for a lifetime. Consistency** is the **key** word. Remember that you can combine aerobic activities. For example, you can take an aerobic dance course that meets twice a week, then go for a brisk pace walk for your third activity. Or for your third activity, you could run in place five minutes, jump rope for three minutes, and dance aerobically for twelve minutes to reach your twenty-minute minimum aerobic program.

Now and then exercise—no matter how enthusiastically engaged in—will not build or maintain fitness. We all have days when we don't feel like exercising. That's normal. Choosing an activity that you like most of the time will help you make exercising on the "down" days less of a chore. Perhaps that is exactly why you chose aerobic dance!

Individualized Programs

As you prepare your program, establish the following guidelines to insure yourself success:

1   Assess fitness in the beginning.

Discuss your plans with your doctor. Sudden exertion could be enough of a shock to your cardiorespiratory system to lead to serious complications. Have a physical examination that gives you a complete understanding of your current health status and that provides guidelines or limitations. (See Chapter 11 for specifics to limitations.) Determine fitness level by means of a stress test (fitness test).

2   Set realistic goals.

Make sure that they are goals you can reach. Write a self-contract covering one month for starters (chart 1 in Appendix). Agree with yourself that you will set aside one hour, three times a week for your aerobic dance program. For many, a beginning level of fitness can be obtained in eight to ten weeks, if all aerobic criteria are used. Give yourself the gift of patience, for fitness will take **time.** It's all worth it, though, and the dividends are many!

3   Plan time on a weekly basis.

There is no undesirable time other than immediately **after** eating. Early morning before breakfast and shower can be a good time. It is too easy to make excuses later in the day as you become caught up in the daily routine of responsibilities. Also, strenuous exercising just before eating will help decrease your appetite. If, however, you like to use aerobic dance to release the stresses of the day, noon time or before the evening meal are other opportune times.

4   Develop your skill at pulse taking.

At the beginning of an aerobic program, learn to take resting, exercising, recovery, and relaxation pulses accurately using one of the six pulsation points. Resting, recovery, and relaxation pulses are most accurate by timing the pulse for at least fifteen seconds (and multiplying by four). Pulse taking during aerobic exercise is most accurate by an immediate count for six or ten seconds (and multiplying by ten or six, respectively).

5   Chart your progress.

"Participants should be given a specific means of assessing physical status and progress. Working heart rate should be measured during peak levels of exercise to ensure that the intensity of activity is within the desired range. Regular measurement of the recovery heart rate will motivate participants by documenting their progress. Failure to progress as measured by this method may indicate the need for more intense activity during the aerobic phase or may signal the presence of other problems."[5]

By monitoring on paper all aspects of your program, you provide a progress report with immediate feedback for yourself. Monitor and chart progress on the following:

- Resting heart rate.
- Heart rates during your program.
- Your weight maintenance, loss, or gain (details and procedures in Chapter 9).
- Your dietary intake (details and procedures in Chapter 10).
- You also may enjoy keeping a log or journal on your stress management and emotional changes. After you complete eight to ten weeks of dancing, list all of your results (see Appendix). This will provide a "bird's-eye view" of your total progress to date!
- Progress on a variety of alternative aerobic programs: using weights and progressions; pace-walking; running; rope jumping; or cycling.

Monitoring the Resting Pulse Rate

One of the two visible signs of **improvement** in heart and lung fitness that you can see happen on paper is a **lowering** of the resting heart rate. A true "resting" heart rate (RsHR) is not taken in a class but when the individual has been at complete rest (i.e., sleeping) for several hours and just awakens. Keep a clock or watch with a second hand next to your bed. When you awaken (without an alarm clock ring), take your pulse for a **full minute** and record that number as your RsHR (or for thirty seconds and multiply by two; or for fifteen seconds and multiply by four). Do this for **five consecutive mornings**, then determine an average (add all RsHR's and divide by five). This is a rather accurate determination of your resting heart rate.

Note: Unusual stress and **illness** (illness is a type of stress) will sharply **raise** the resting heart rate from previous readings. You will understand why it is so important, then, for normally healthy individuals to find a **positive outlet** for stress, for it affects you even as you sleep (constant rapid heart rate), at a time when the heart ideally should "take a break" and slow down for six to eight hours.

Use chart 6 in the Appendix for recording your resting heart rate. The first week, take five consecutive daily readings, and record this as your initial RsHR. Record your RsHR twice a week thereafter until the conclusion of the eight-to-ten-week course. Record your final reading below your initial reading and determine the loss or gain in RsHR for the eight-to-ten-week period. Also record this RsHR number on chart 8 as a reference and guideline for use during your class monitoring.

Because the RsHR is the basic "thermometer of fitness," after a ten-to-fifteen-week aerobic dance course you may experience similar results as those gathered from other students:

- An average − 3 heartbeats per minute resting heart rate decline.
- An average − 10 heartbeats per minute recorded by "smokers" who quit (or significantly change their consumption) during the course, with as much as a − 24 heartbeats per minute decline recorded recently![6]

Monitoring and Charting During Various Segments of An Aerobic Dance Session

USING CHART 8

Initially (usually for the first two weeks), readings are taken **after every type of exertion** (exercise) so that the individual develops an accurate skill of reading the pulse.

1   Pre-Activity Pulse Rate

According to what you've just been doing prior to class, this reading will greatly vary from day to day and from individual to individual. Take this reading on your **own** for six seconds, add a zero, and record. It will give you a starting point for this session.

2   After the Warm-Up Dance

The warm-up dance will demand a stretching pace or tempo now and will be higher than the pre-activity pulse rate. Taking this pulse rate will clearly demonstrate that a **stretching routine** to music is also **NOT aerobic**—the heart rate will not be in the training zone. If you are in the training zone already from only stretching, you can see that you are either really out of shape or have limitations. It will clearly demonstrate to you that your "aerobic" dancing will have to be performed in "intervals" for you to keep up for a twenty-minute (plus) duration. Take your pulse for six seconds, add a zero, and record.

3   After the Warm-Up Jog or Jumping Rope

This warm-up conclusion transitional aerobic activity is included to fully get your heart rate up to the training zone. Your jog/rope jumping pace must be one in which you can endure for three to five minutes of background music, or of a song being played. If you can carry on a conversation with someone or sing the tune, it is the right pace. Don't run all-out and then walk. Find a pace that you can endure the entire time. Try jogging or jumping rope to the beat of the music (or every other beat), if you are **"fit."** Perform jogging or jumping to every other beat of the music in thirty-second intervals to start, if you are "unfit" and **conditioning.**

4   Immediate Count During and/or After an Aerobic Dance Interval

As you are beginning a conditioning aerobic dance program, you'll want to monitor your pace every several minutes, or after each song so that you can develop the skill of constant endurance pacing. This will lead up to your continual dancing for twenty to thirty minutes of the aerobic dance gesture and step pattern movements or routines.

When you take a pulse rate during the learning process and find that your pace is **below** your established "training zone," do **more** work, or increase your intensity. If you are recording a pulse rate **higher** than your established "training zone," do **less** work, or lower your intensity. Continuing at a pace that is too intensive will prove to be an "anaerobic" exercise program—too much immediately followed by too little (you must recover and catch your breath). This yo-yo pace is **not** aerobic conditioning, so try for the constant pacing suggested previously.

The pulse-monitoring procedure during aerobic dance is to slow down and walk, find your pulse, and count it for either **six, ten, or fifteen seconds.** Each of these counts has been found to be a scientifically accurate measurement for aerobic activity pulse rates. Once you (or your instructor) determine whether you will count for six, ten, or fifteen seconds **directly following aerobic dance, multiply the number you get times ten** if using the six-second count, **times six** if using a ten-second count, or **times four** if using a fifteen-second count. **Each of these newly multiplied numbers will equal heartbeats per minute**, and hopefully will be in your training zone!

Note: It is found to be easiest to take a six-second count, for all you do is "add a zero" to what pulse you feel and record that number. Persons must carefully begin and end exactly with a timer. Taking the immediate count during/after aerobic dance using a timed count of greater than fifteen seconds will tend to be inaccurate, since the heart rate slows down to a "recovery" pulse rather rapidly.

Also, you will soon recognize that as your cardiorespiratory system becomes more fit or efficient, work (exercise) will become easier, and you will be forced to increase the intensity of your activities by using larger arm movements, lifting your knees higher, hopping more, etc. By using the training zone, you automatically compensate for this increased fitness and still maintain the same training effect.

The count just mentioned is recorded as the "I", or immediate count taken during/after a dance and is recorded as such on the aforementioned chart. This count should **always** be in the training zone and doesn't fluctuate.

Since once you start and **never** completely stop or sit down until the latter part of the hour, **do not sit down to record**—simply bend over with a hamstring stretch, record, and keep walking. You do not want to encourage varicose veins, so keep moving!

5   Recovery Heart Rate Count, One Minute After

The recovery heart rate count, or "R" on the charting, is taken **one minute after** the previously monitored count (the "immediate" training zone count). This will visually show you on paper how your heart is recovering from strenuous exercise and is the **second measure of fitness that you can see happen on paper.** As you become more physically fit, the recovery count will get down lower and lower **away from** the immediate training zone count. This, then, is the reason for the count—so you can see your fitness improving on paper before your very eyes! It also provides a brief recovery interval to catch your breath for the **conditioning** dancer.

6   After the Cool-Down Exercises/Routine

This is only taken the first several weeks to show the new dancer how the heart responds to getting back to the pre-activity pulse count at which he or she started. This count should be **lower** than 120 beats per minute. Do not leave an hour or session of exercise with a higher heart rate. Lie on the floor another minute or two and retake the count until it comes down. Because you'll experience a concluding activity of relaxation, this count is eliminated after the first two weeks, and a count is taken only after relaxation at the end of the hour or session.

7   After Strength Training

If a pulse is taken during the strength training phase,

you will discover this is **not** an aerobic activity. According to your exertion, it would be clearly above or markedly below your training zone.

"To prevent muscle imbalance, specific exercises **should be** used to strengthen the antagonists to those muscles used forcefully and repetitively during aerobic exercise. Dance exercise does little to strengthen either the **abdominal** muscles or the muscles that **dorsiflex the foot.** Specific strengthening of these muscles is important to avoid the potentially imbalancing effects of dance exercise."[7]

8 After Relaxation

In concluding the hour, a final count is taken to visually show the dancer several significant happenings. First, the heart rate may very well be **lower** than when the individual began the hour even with **only** three minutes of relaxation! And the individual will find that he or she, with a conscious effort to train the mind to relaxation, can get the heart rate down very close, if not to, each individual's **resting** heart rate!

Relaxation heart rates achieved in class in contrast to resting heart rates taken at home in bed after six to eight hours of sleep revealed the following results recently:

After just three minutes of relaxation technique following an intense aerobic dance workout, students were able to achieve heart rates which were, on an average, **three beats lower than their average resting heart rates recorded after six to eight hours of sleep!**[8]

Enjoyment Is Found Through Variety

Insure the success of this activity by having a program with variety and one in which you totally enjoy participating. Variety would include using all of the principles and possibilities in choreography (Chapter 8) and choosing a wide selection of music.

Choose the Best Location

Select a convenient and physiologically safe location for your program. Choose a **wood**-based floor or an area carpeted with flat nap and thick padding. Try not to exercise on concrete, since there is no "give" or buoyancy to it. Concrete adds unnecessary stress on your legs and feet.

"A resilient floor should be selected for exercise that involves repeated foot impacts. If such a surface is not available, the exercise routines should be modified to ensure that the feet remain close to the floor throughout the program."[9]

Select Proper Clothing

Choosing what to wear for the environment in which you are dancing is quite important. Safety, comfort, and ease of movement are the keys for aerobic dance apparel. Dress in layers. A warm-up sweatsuit or jogging suit will assist in increasing the temperature of your arm and leg muscles during the warm-up portion of the hour. On very warm, or highly humid and warm days, this, of course, is unnecessary. Select cotton material over others since it absorbs perspiration better than other fabrics. When cotton clothing becomes damp, the surrounding air causes the moisture to evaporate, and this will cool your body.

During the dance routines, you want to be free to move in all directions and sweat freely, so wear as little as possible, especially when the temperature and relative humidity are high.

Long, loose slacks should be avoided, as they can catch under the feet. Tight-fitting garments should be avoided, as they restrict flexibility. The best advice for someone vigorously exercising is to keep clothing to a comfortable minimum. This allows unrestricted motion and facilitates loss of excessive body heat.[10]

Possibilities are shorts and a tee shirt, a leotard (and tights, but the tights **only** in cold weather), newly designed cotton exercise body suits, or—for women—shorts and a swimsuit with bra support for full-figured persons.

Wear proper-fitting cotton socks to help keep your feet free from blisters and to keep your feet drier. Underclothing needs to give you good support. Jockey shorts or, better yet, an athletic supporter for men and a bra that fits snugly and holds firmly for women, are important. In regards to bra support, there is a detailed section of related information in Chapter 11, for those who have this special concern.

Just be sure that you do not wear too much clothing and get overheated. Persons very overweight or obese are especially prime targets for overheating because they have a thick layer of fat tissue between internal organs and the outside layer of skin. It works like insulation and keeps internal heat in. This means that the internal body systems may overheat and cause heat exhaustion or heat stroke. So don't try to "sweat" water pounds off by wearing lots of clothing or rubber-lined sweatsuits. Sweat and water loss are your cooling mechanisms and are **not** to be used as a measurement for weight loss (for water is **not** fat!). A section on what **not** to wear is included in Chapter 11.

Buy the Proper Shoes

Appropriate, well-constructed shoes for this activity are a must! They will insure not only your comfort, but also will help prevent injuries (i.e., achilles tendon strain, heel bruises), particularly if all of this is new to you. You will find that this investment is well worth your attention—the dividends will pay off very soon after you begin your program. The following are guidelines when selecting an appropriate aerobic dance shoe. In order of importance:

1
Select a shoe that is designed to take the stress of repeated shock to the knees, lower legs, ankles, and feet. You **must** have a shoe that has a lot of spongy cushioning in the arch and rubber on the heel. In other words, wear a shoe with thick rubber soles!

2
Do not select a wide heel flair (of rubber) if you have the tendency toward pronated ankles (lower leg bones do not sit directly on the ankle). This (heel flair) will not only limit, to some degree, your lateral (sideward) movement, but also it will not provide the appropriate correction to avoid future possible injury to naturally weak ankles, as it does in jogging—which is all forward movement. Pronation of ankles can best be corrected **inside** the shoe by means of:

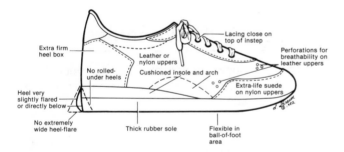

Figure 2-1.

- Raising the arch with a specifically designed wedge.
- Controlling the floor contact of various portions of the foot by means of a specially designed orthotic (prescribed corrective device for the foot).
- An **extra firm** heel box.

If you do not have pronated ankles, also purposefully

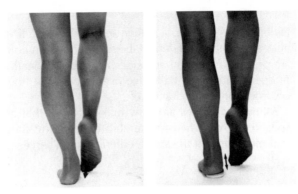

Figure 2-2. Left: Pronation. Right: Correction with a sports orthotic.

select a rubber heel with no wide flair but one that is directly below the heel, or flairs only slightly to provide ease in executing the various sideward moves.

3
Try this on the shoe you're thinking of buying or using: bend the shoe in half (sole out) so that the toe is placed inside the heel. If the shoe bends, wear it. If the shoe doesn't bend very well, it will be an inflexible shoe in which to dance. You want foot flexibility while you move, especially in the ball of the foot area of the shoe.

"During aerobic dance, most impacts are made on the balls of the feet, so the shoes worn should have good cushioning in that location."[11]

4
Lacing should be of the style that has five or six eyelets **closely** spaced on the top of the instep. Wide lacing from the base of your toes across the entire instep will provide less support for lateral movement. This type of shoe (canvas "low-tops") may tend to make your foot roll outward, causing ankle twisting or a sprain.

5
The sole of the shoe should have a relatively smooth tread[12] and should be of white rubber, designed for aerobic dance or court use. Jogging shoes with black rubber soles, designed for road and track running and with rubber triangles, squares, circles, or thick waves provide excellent **forward** movement, but since aerobic dance consists of forward, backward, and lateral movement, this is not a best choice of shoe sole.

"The rough treads of most running shoes can be hazardous during aerobic dance exercise as they can cause the feet to come to an abrupt halt each time they strike the floor. Thus, most shoes designed for running are unsuitable for aerobic dance."[13]

6

Nylon uppers are cooler than leather uppers. If an all-leather shoe is preferred, be sure ventilation holes are present on the top and sides. Extra design leather or suede along the ball-edge of the foot area (toes) provides for a longer shoe life.

Many companies are now making shoes that are specifically designed for aerobic dance. Any shoes that meet most of the above criteria should serve you well.

Develop Associated Regular Habits: Eating/Sleeping/ Relaxing

In order to provide the fuel needed to produce the energy required for aerobic dance ("going"), and to insure proper body regulatory functions, growth, and repair ("growing"), eat a well-balanced diet that provides all the nutrients you need to stay well and be able to perform well (see Chapter 10).

Refrain from eating for one, or preferably two, hours before participating in aerobic activity. **Eat afterwards.** With the digestion of food, an increased amount of blood and oxygen is needed in the digestive tract. With exercise, as much as 100 times more oxygen is needed in the working muscles, i.e., arms and legs, than when at rest. Your body will just have great difficulty supplying an increase in blood and oxygen to two major body functions at once!

Establish quality time for proper relaxation and adequate sleep. These are important restorative mechanisms. Since aerobic dance will increase your energy level, the body's way of restoring energy ("energizing" you) is through relaxation and sleep. These also help to restore the ability to concentrate and to maintain a positive attitude and self-confidence. Physiologically, relaxation and sleep help by lowering both the body temperature and heart rate, which, in turn, lower the body's demand for oxygen and nutrients. These conserve, while restoring, the body's supply of energy.

Incorporate Proper Exercise Habits

1   Breathing Technique

Breathe continuously. Your entire system, especially your working muscles, **constantly need oxygen.** Hol-

ding your breath and turning red is **never** an appropriate way to exercise. While performing the warm-up and cool-down stretching (or any strengthening exercise), **exhale** when you **stretch**, and **inhale** when you **relax** your muscles. Cue yourself: "breathe out and stretch," "breathe in and relax." (See Chapters 4, 6, and 7 for more specifics on breathing.)

2   Fluid Intake

Frequent small intakes of fluid throughout your day is best. For complete details on water intake, see Chapter 11.

3   Missing A While?

Return to aerobic dance slowly. If for any reason you miss activity several times, you will need to start more cautiously as though beginning a new program.

For example, you may have a bout of flu and are then unable to exercise for a week. When you are able to exercise again, do **not** plan to start where you left off. You will need to return cautiously to the fitness level that you were at before illness. Dr. Lenore Zohlman, a leading cardiologist in the United States, has stated that after just five weeks you will lose approximately half of your fitness program gains if you discontinue your program totally. And, after ten weeks of no aerobic activity, you will have lost most of the fitness gains that you experienced.[14] So realize this physiological phenomenon and return slowly and systematically whenever a circumstance curtails your program.

Consider the Variables

There are numerous variables to be considered and planned for when engaging in an aerobic dance program. A few are:

- The environmental temperature.
- The relative humidity.
- Physiological changes with the menstrual cycle.
- Illness, infection, or injury present.
- The amount of negative stress you are currently experiencing.

All of these variables will make changes in how your body responds during an aerobic dance program. Be flexible in your program when any new factor enters into the picture and change your procedure accordingly.

1

Above 85° F. room or outside temperature, never aerobic dance—go aerobic swim in an air-conditioned environment.

2

A high relative humidity combined with a hot day are two good reasons to, again, aerobic swim in an air-conditioned environment. (You can develop heat stress even in an outside pool in a hot and humid environment. The key is the **cool** air temperature.)

3

For many women, the menstrual cycle creates no new concerns. Practicing good habits of physical fitness and nutrition[15] are the best words of advice to alleviate any temporary discomforts experienced. (Refer to Chapter 11 for more details.)

4

The presence of illness, infection, or injury will show up in your "thermometer" of fitness—your pulse. It will be higher at rest and will escalate to the training zone with less than your usual effort. So take it easy and decide whether to mentally "walk" through your program to maintain your discipline of exercising, or to just curtail exercise until you're well again.

5

Negative stress, like illness, will escalate your heart rate **at rest or during aerobic dancing.** You, again, will have to closely monitor your heart rate to keep it at your training zone so that you don't overtax your heart. (More on stress-related information in Chapter 7.)

Other variables to be considered are the presence of various temporary limitations, or injury-related concerns. A complete discussion on these areas can be found in Chapter 11.

Aerobic Dance—A New Release from Stress

The natural tranquilizer—routine exercise.

Because we are all victims of unwanted daily pressures, we all find a way to release these pressures. Some ways are good for our health and some are detrimental. But what we must recognize is that we all do **something** to release the stress and tensions in our lives! It is the way we maintain our mental balance—the way in which we cope with life. Some

people smoke, some drink alcohol, or coffee, or soda pop to excess, others eat to excess, some play loud music or bang out a few tunes on a musical instrument, some chew gum wildly—the list is endless! Some habits are harmless; some are harmful.

If you don't like the way you look and feel—if you're too fat, too lean and weak, too out of breath doing any daily activities, are listless, or bored, then try allowing aerobic dance to assist you in alleviating that unwanted stress. Using aerobic dance as your **stress release** will give you a healthy outlet for all those problems or situations or pressures that you accumulate. You can get so turned on to aerobic dance that at the end of a session, you can pick up those cares that you put aside for a few moments and charge into them with renewed vigor! Life is situations and life is change. How we each adapt to and cope with these situations or changes reveals our true human quality. So, forget all those unhealthy crutches you've established as **habits of choice** to relieve the stress in your life!

1 Smoking

Smoking tobacco causes the lung capillaries to decrease in size (constrict), which, in turn, restricts the ability of your cardiorespiratory system to circulate the needed oxygen to your body parts. When you are performing an activity that requires the use of more oxygen, why would you want to compound the situation by **choosing** to allow less oxygen supply and use to take place?

Fortunately, more and more individuals who enroll in aerobic dance courses are not inclined to smoke cigarettes. Recent findings show that 88 percent of the students who enroll in aerobic dance do not smoke cigarettes.[16]

2 Alcohol

Try to abstain from the use of the number one drug problem— alcohol. Alcohol causes a constriction of the coronary arteries supplying the heart at the same time your exercise program is demanding an **increase** of oxygen from the heart. Again, why **choose** to allow less oxygen and nutrient supply to occur when you need more? Kick the habit and get "hooked" on aerobic dance instead. If you do drink, do so in moderation after exercising or at least four hours before you aerobic dance. And then work at a decreased intensity level. The two activities—drinking followed by aerobic dancing—simply do not go together.

3 Overeating

Consuming far too much food is a habit by **choice** that all too many Americans engage in today. Chapters 9 and 10 contain an extensive discussion on this topic, since it is one of the **primary** reasons why people begin aerobic dancing. Eighty-two percent of all the individuals who enroll in an aerobic dance course specifically state that they desire to lose fat weight.[17]

If one of your goals is fat weight loss (or lean weight gain), specific program adjustments must be made, for this text is primarily designed to develop and maintain heart and lung fitness. Altering your basic program to accommodate other important goals is possible. You simply need to **know the principles involved to obtain the results you desire.**

4 Caffeine

Like nicotine, caffeine has immediate effects on blood pressure. The equivalent of two or three cups of coffee raises blood pressure of normal people an average of 14/10 points—enough to bring many of them into the range of "mild" hypertension. [18] Since hypertension is a risk factor for heart disease, moderation seems to be the best avenue when it comes to caffeine.

Evaluate Your Progress and Program

Review the monitored data you've been collecting on yourself. Correct any problem areas you can determine. It may seem remarkable how one fun-filled activity can create so much positive change for the better in most individuals.

A Review Checklist

Go through the following to be sure you've tried your best to plan and execute a top-notch program for yourself.

- Assess fitness in the very beginning.
- Set realistic goals.
- Plan time on a weekly basis.
- Develop your skill at pulse taking.
- Chart your progress:
  - Monitoring resting pulse rate.
  - Monitoring various segments of the aerobic dance session
  - Weight maintenance/loss/gain.

- Dietary intake.
- Journal on stress management adjustments or emotional change
- Enjoyment is found through variety.
- Choose the best location.
- Select proper clothing to wear.
- Buy the proper shoes for this unique activity.
- Develop associated regular habits: eating/sleeping/relaxing.
- Incorporate proper exercise habits: breathing technique/fluid intake/missing activity/and beginning again.
- Consider the variables: temperature/relative humidity/menstrual cycle/illness, infection, or injury/presence of negative stress.
- Allow aerobic dance to become your new release from stress: Forget smoking/alcohol/overeating/excessive caffeine.
- Evaluate your progress and your program.

Keep Dancing— Keep Smiling—Keep Fit

You have completed your aerobic dance program preparation, and now you are ready to begin! Many people who have been habitual dropouts from other fitness programs are now enthusiastic and dedicated members of aerobic dance programs. The combination of music, dance, and the social atmosphere can become irresistible. Having the basic step and gesture patterns enumerated and designed into an easy learning and recall format (as is presented in this text) will provide you with a foundation from which your program can take off in many creative possibilities. It is hoped that you will consider aerobic dance so much fun and so beneficial that you will be involved for life!

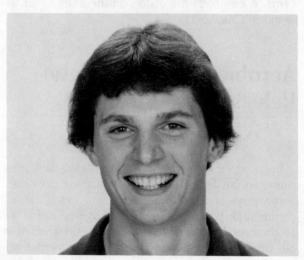

Figure 2-3.

3

POSTURE:
Your Program Begins Here!

Why Include Posture?

Probably the key reason to include posture information in an aerobic dance course is to **save your back**! In order to insure that you are performing exercises in the **safest** possible fashion, you must understand good postural techniques, regardless of the activity you're performing. Developing good postural habits will insure that **your spine is always held in a stabilized manner.**

Understanding the Mechanics

The downward pressure of gravity applied to the bones of the upright, balanced skeleton will tend to cause it to buckle at three principal points: hip, knee, and ankle. And, since the weight of the body is largely in front of the spinal column, the body will tend to fall forward. To counteract these tendencies toward buckling and falling forward, we have five muscles, or muscle groups, which are designed to be "anti-gravity" in nature and which allow for an upright, balanced skeleton. Figure 3-3 shows these muscles and their relationship to the upright skeleton. These "anti-gravity" muscle groups that are responsible for holding us erect are located in the:

● Back, along the spinal column.
● Abdomen.
● Buttocks.

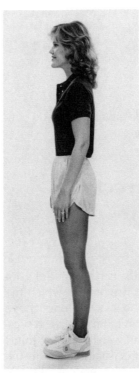

Figure 3-1.

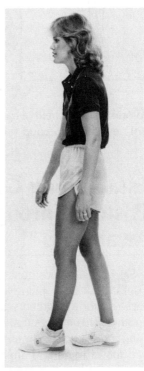

Figure 3-2.

● Front of the thighs.
● Calves.

To develop good posture, the position of the spine, pelvic girdle, and hip joints (which act as the main hinges of the body) need to be controlled, and is done

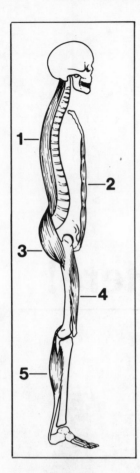

Figure 3-3.

so primarily by the five muscle groups. **How** you control determines a **good** posture.

Establishing Correct Posture Through Awareness

Safe, efficient positions for the performance of exercise and all daily living tasks are ones in which the various body segments are balanced—one above another. This insures that a minimum of uneven pressure and friction occurs in the weight-bearing joints and that a minimum amount of strain occurs in the adjoining muscles, ligaments, and tendons. Initially in the learning process, you need to develop a kinesthetic awareness (sensation of position, movement, tension, etc., of parts of the body) so that you feel uncomfortable when moving through tasks incorrectly or inefficiently (i.e., while using poor posture). As you then develop continual good postural awareness, you will begin to move in well-aligned positions automatically!

This awareness will also provide you with a margin for safety in each joint, so that an unexpected force won't immediately push the joint beyond its normal limits and cause injury. And when your body is in proper alignment, it is in the best, most efficient position to resist the downward pull of gravity with the least amount of negative stress and effort. **A balanced posture makes full and efficient use of the force of gravity (by aligning all parts) so that the pull is directly downward through the supporting parts.** This allows the muscles to do minimal work in maintaining the body in an erect position. The ligaments and muscles surrounding each joint hold the part in place, cooperating with the pull of gravity instead of constantly having to work against it. Efficiency is thus obtained.

Balanced Static/ Dynamic Postures

A balanced standing posture is established by having:

1
The head and **stretched** neck balanced on top of the spine and centered above the shoulders, keeping your chin parallel to the floor.

2
Your shoulders pulled **back** and **down** (in a relaxed position).

3
Your chest and rib cage raised **up**.

4
Your abdominal muscles pulled **in and up**, under the rib cage.

5
The pelvic girdle pulled **down and under**, tightening the buttocks. The pelvis rests on the two thigh bones balanced over two arched feet.

6
Your knees **relaxed.** Locking your knees in a hyperextended position causes imbalance and makes you more susceptible to knee injury.

7
Your weight distributed equally on both feet while standing with feet **parallel** and toes pointing forward as you take the weight on the **outer** half of the feet.

8
Your arms **relaxed.**

SIDE VIEW

Line of gravity passes:
1. Tip of ear
2. Center of shoulders
3. Slightly behind center of hip
4. Behind knee cap
5. In front of ankle joint
6. Body line perpendicular through weight center

BACK VIEW

Line of gravity passes:
1. Through mid-head
2. Mid-trunk
3. Mid-waist
4. Mid-ankle

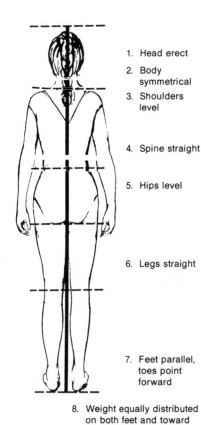

1. Head up

2. Chin parallel to floor

3. Ear above middle of shoulder

4. Tip of shoulder over hip joint

5. Shoulders relaxed and down

6. Chest and rib cage lifted; "easy"

7. Abdomen flat

8. Pelvis balanced; front of pelvis and thigh in a continuous line

9. Knees unlocked or slightly flexed; "easy"

10. Feet parallel, body weight centered between heel and toe and carried on outer half of feet

1. Head erect

2. Body symmetrical

3. Shoulders level

4. Spine straight

5. Hips level

6. Legs straight

7. Feet parallel, toes point forward

8. Weight equally distributed on both feet and toward outer half of each foot

Figure 3-4. Good Postures.

The above key positions apply to standing. If each body segment is balanced, a vertical line should extend from the tip of the ear through the center of the shoulder, slightly behind center of hip, behind the kneecap, and just in front of the ankle joint. Whenever one part moves out of this line (as shown in Figure 3-4), your center of gravity shifts in the **direction** of that movement, and another part of you must then adjust in the opposite direction in order to maintain the center of gravity back over your base of support. Keeping this in mind will assist you in establishing the balancing, or "correct postural awareness," mentioned earlier to enable you to move well in any position and direction you choose—be they stationary moves like lunges and widestride varieties, or dynamic moves like rocking or jogging.

Poor Posture—A Habit That Can Be Changed

If any segment is out of body alignment, your weight distribution will be uneven over your base of support and will put unnecessary strain on muscles, bones, and joints. This will soon cause fatigue.

Poor posture is very definitely a habit that can be changed, but it will take time, since the habit that you now have has been a part of you for a long time. Since most muscles are in pairs, if a muscle is constantly shortened, its opposing muscle will lengthen and become weak from disuse. Therefore, stretching (lengthening) one set of muscles, while simultaneously contracting (shortening) the opposing set of mus-

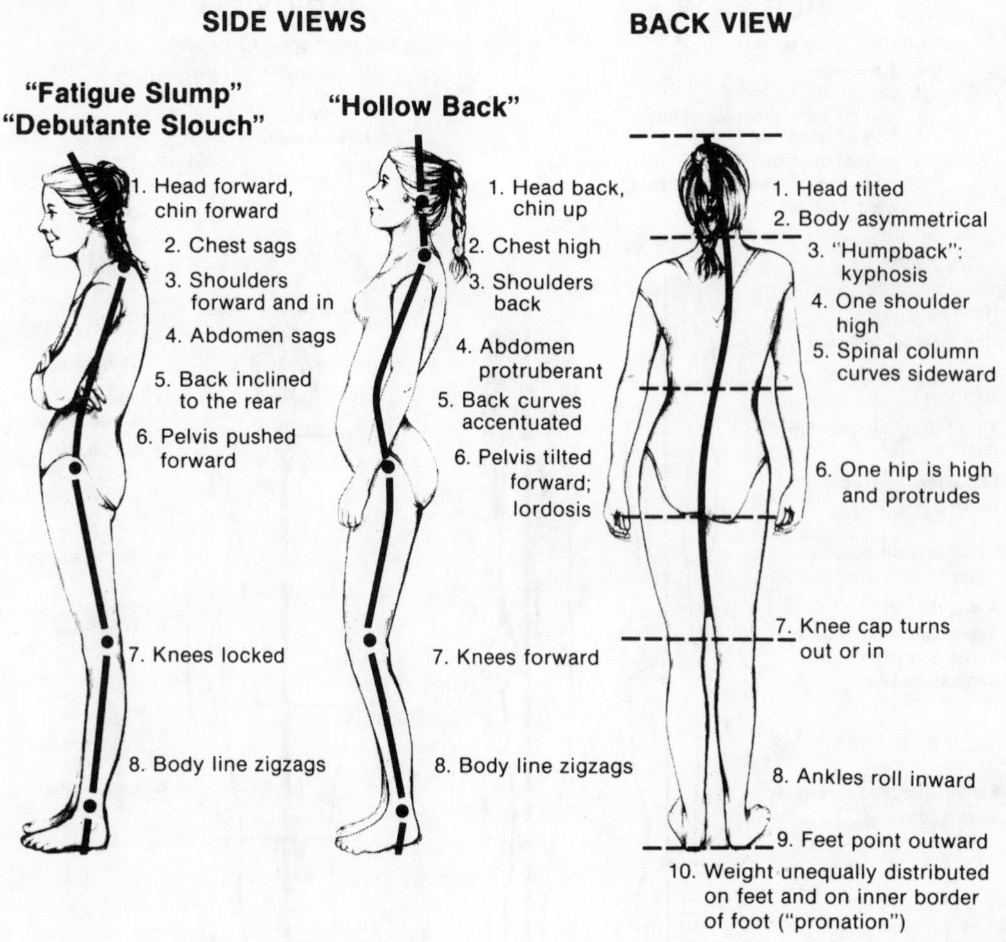

SIDE VIEWS   **BACK VIEW**

"Fatigue Slump"
"Debutante Slouch"   "Hollow Back"

1. Head forward, chin forward
2. Chest sags
3. Shoulders forward and in
4. Abdomen sags
5. Back inclined to the rear
6. Pelvis pushed forward
7. Knees locked
8. Body line zigzags

1. Head back, chin up
2. Chest high
3. Shoulders back
4. Abdomen protruberant
5. Back curves accentuated
6. Pelvis tilted forward; lordosis
7. Knees forward
8. Body line zigzags

1. Head tilted
2. Body asymmetrical
3. "Humpback": kyphosis
4. One shoulder high
5. Spinal column curves sideward
6. One hip is high and protrudes
7. Knee cap turns out or in
8. Ankles roll inward
9. Feet point outward
10. Weight unequally distributed on feet and on inner border of foot ("pronation")

Figure 3-5. Poor Postures.

cles, **and then repeating vice versa**, will strengthen both (especially if additional weight resistance is used). With this thought in mind, you can understand why stretching and strengthening your muscles will develop an improved posture. For if your body is to move freely, every muscle needs to be able to shorten or lengthen in either a strong, quick manner or a slow, relaxed manner. Chapters 4 and 6 include stretching and strength training and will therefore assist you further in understanding and obtaining your good posture goals.

Efficient Positions

If you now exhibit poor posture during aerobic dance movement activities, you will need to re-educate your neuromuscular system. This will take patience, persistence, and a sincere desire on your part to want to improve both your appearance and the efficiency of your body.

If you were born free from hereditary or congenital deformities, you **can** obtain good posture! It's all a matter of:

- Understanding balanced postures.
- Developing a kinesthetic awareness of your body positions during all movement.
- Developing strong and yet relaxed muscles, and flexible joints.
- Desiring to obtain good posture.
- Discipline to continue what you have learned.

As you understand correct technique, challenge yourself to try using these positions for every phase of your program, i.e., stretching, aerobic dancing, and strength training exercises.

At first you'll be "thinking through" the activity, but with persistent practice and desire, you can exchange any former faulty habits for safe, more complimentary ones.

Standing

Stationary Purposes: If you can exhibit the balanced standing posture described and pictured earlier for activities that require a **stationary**, poised, controlled look, you've mastered this area already!

Dynamic Purposes: Performing the aerobic dance gesture and step patterns will require you to exhibit a different body position, or posture, than when you are just standing stationary and poised. These are the times when you are **preparing to move dynamically— in some direction through space** (forward, backward, laterally, up, down, etc.). While preparing to move through space, the broader your base of support, the lower your center of gravity (weight center) becomes. This, then, allows for better balance so that you can move quickly and more efficiently in any direction.

Developing Your Postural Awareness Through Posture Exercises

Exercising the anti-gravity muscles is a fundamental part of any general conditioning program. In order to develop and then maintain a good posture, these muscles need to be:

- **Strong** enough to perform their functions.
- **Flexible** enough to allow a variety of movement.
- **Relaxed** enough to perform with ease.

Therefore, establishing a program of strength exercises (as found in Chapter 6) for the abdomen, lower back, hip, thigh, and calf areas will help you to obtain a balanced pelvic alignment and provide the means for efficient and painless movement. And, as mentioned, each joint involved needs to be flexible enough to permit the full range of movement possible from these groups of anti-gravity muscles so that any new position can be properly maintained. The exercises in this chapter (and in Chapter 4) will help you to develop joint flexibility of the anti-gravity muscle groups needed to maintain correct postures. And establishing a program of relaxation (see Chapter 7) will assist with ease of performance, while moving or while motionless.

However, the **best** exercise that you can do for yourself is both a physical and mental one: **Become aware of correct postural technique with every move you make.** Then practice this physical and mental conditioning constantly until it becomes a habit—until it becomes you.

Note: Review the eight key cues for establishing good posture (i.e., chest up, shoulders down, etc.) and then proceed with the following exercises:

Elbows Wide 'N Close

To understand the awareness of "space between shoulder blades" **contracted** and then **widely stretched**, keeping chest raised in either direction:

1
Clasp your hands loosely behind your head. Keep your **elbows out and high**, shoulders down and chin parallel to the floor. **4 counts.**

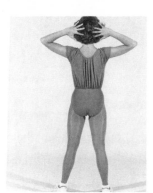

Figure 3-6.

2
Do not tightly lace fingers **behind the neck.** Pulling on the cervical spine is not a good body position technique.

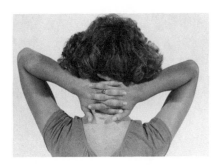

Figure 3-7.

3
Exhale, and widen the space between your shoulder blades by bringing elbows **together** in front of your nose. **Hold. 4 counts.**

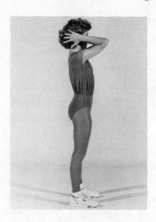

Figure 3-8.

4

Inhale, and return elbows **wide** to the sides (Figure 3-8). **4 counts.**

5

Exhale and pull your elbows **up and back**, tightly contracting the space between your shoulder blades. Hold. **4 counts.**

6

Inhale and return **elbows wide** to the sides (Figure 3-6). **4 counts.**

7

For variety, repeat attempting to touch elbows together, first **in front of forehead** and **below the chin**, maintaining the good posture position.

Cues: Elbows out and high, together, wide, up and back, wide.

Rotater Cuff Exercise

To develop free movement of shoulder joints:

1

Stand in correct alignment with lowered arms, **cross** your wrists in front of you, palms down, wrists clenched. **4 counts.**

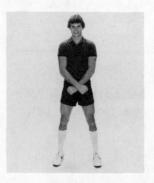

Figure 3-9.

2

In this position, **raise** your arms forward and above your head, fists now facing out and wrists still **crossed. 4 counts.**

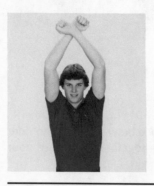

Figure 3-10.

3

Open your arms **wide**, fists down **and lower** them in a circle to starting position with wrists crossed in front of you. **4 counts.**

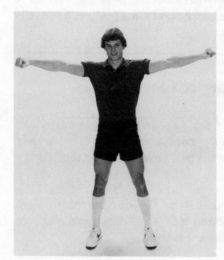

Figure 3-11.

4

Repeat slowly 4 times. **48 counts.**

Note: Don't hunch your shoulders—keep them down throughout movement.

Cues: Cross, raise crossed, open-wide, and lower.

Rib Lifter

To establish the awareness to the all-important position of "chest high" (and not sagging), this exercise will help to isolate and stretch the intercostal (rib) muscles:

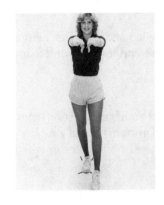
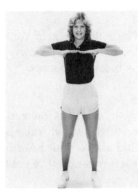

1

Stand in correct alignment, with your **arms forward** and **parallel** to the ground. Place your thumbs and index fingers of each hand together, hands forward, palms down. **4 counts.**

2

Bend your elbows, bring your arms back, and place your palms parallel to the ground above your breast, with your **thumbs** snugly **under the armpits** and elbows held wide and parallel to the ground. **4 counts.**

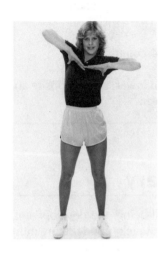

3

Without lifting your shoulders or bending forward, **lift your entire rib section as high as you can.** Breathe deeply, inhale and exhale. **8 counts.**

4

Now **lift** your elbow high **and stretch** rib cage on one side.   **4 counts.**

5

Lower raised elbow to shoulder level. **4 counts.**

6

Repeat with lifting and lowering of other elbow. **8 counts.**

7

Repeat **raising both** together; **lower. 8 counts.**

Cues: Stand; thumbs under armpits; lift ribs and breathe; lift and stretch, lower; repeat other side; repeat both.

Reaching Correctly

To establish the awareness in keeping the **shoulders back and down** as you perform arm movement that is forward and upward:

1

Stand in correct alignment. Place the back of your left hand on your central lower back and pelvic girdle area. **4 counts.**

2

Slowly **raise** your right arm forward and in front of your body above your head, keeping your lower arm and hand straight and your elbow flexed. **4 counts.**

3

Slowly **lower** your arm to its original position in standing alignment. **4 counts.**

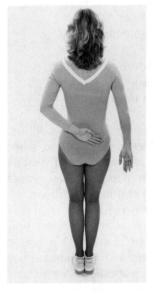
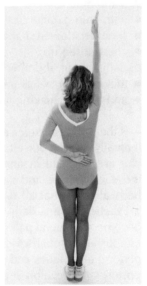

Figure 3-15.   **Figure 3-16.**

4

Place the back of your right hand on your central lower back, and slowly **raise and lower** your left arm as before. **8 counts.**

5

With both arms lowered and both hands resting lightly on thighs, slowly **raise both arms** in front of your body and above your head in the same manner in which each was raised. **4 counts.**

6

Slowly **lower** to original position. **4 counts.**

7

Repeat all, once again. **24 counts.**

Cues: Stand; raise one and lower; raise opposite and lower; raise both and lower.

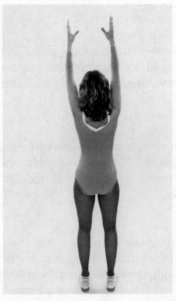

Figure 3-17.

Posture Summary

For your total daily well-being, the development, continued awareness, and usage of good posture must become important enough to you to be a life-long endeavor. So start now! Are you sitting correctly while reading how to improve your posture? Think good posture at all times!

The knowledge of a well-aligned body and the development of a kinesthetic awareness (feeling) of good posture are the first steps toward acquiring good postural habits. This constant awareness of good posture—

- Standing tall
- with chin parallel to the floor
- shoulders lowered and pulled back tight
- chest raised up
- pulling your abdomen first in and then up
- tucking your pelvis under
- and thereby making your torso erect

—is the one best exercise that you can physically and mentally do for yourself. **Then remember, too, when you are engaged in any exercise program, that to move efficiently and safely depends upon proper body alignment at all times and in all positions.**

Practicing on a daily basis is required for this to become an integral part of you. Good posture is only established through **discipline**. Setting aside time to perform techniques and exercises to encourage good posture and develop strength and flexibility, accompanied by constant attention to posture throughout your daily living tasks, will make this all become a reality to you. You can improve as you move—all day, every day—for this is where your total program for a fit figure, or physique, begins!

The following is an index review of all of the posture exercises which were described in this chapter, in the order in which they were presented:

- Elbows Wide 'N Close
- Rotator Cuff Exercise
- Rib Lifter
- Reaching Correctly

4

THE WARM-UP:
A Catalogue of Exercises and A Routine

Function of the Warm-Up

The initial phase of an exercise session is entitled "the warm-up" because that is exactly what the entire body slowly experiences—a gradual **increase in body temperature** accompanied by the various needed physiological changes. The warm-up will prepare you for the strenuous activities of your program yet to come, because it:

- Provides a **gradual** increase in the intensity of the work (or stress) that you place on your heart.
- Promotes circulation by beginning the process of delivering more oxygen and nutrients to the working muscles.
- Prepares your muscles, tendons, ligaments, and joints for a safe, comfortable, more injury-free activity hour.
- Increases your range of motion so that you can do more work.
- Tends to reduce muscle soreness (if **static** stretching is performed).
- Develops a unique kinesthetic awareness of each muscle group being toned.
- Provides the time needed for the mental transition from your daily stressors to total involvement in your physical workout and stress-release program.

With so many advantages you'll never want to skip this vital portion of your total aerobic dance program.

Benefits in Detail

A list of benefits derived from the warm-up were just enumerated. Here is a look at each in detail:

1

The most important reason to include a warm-up in your workout program is to provide a **gradual** increase in the intensity of the work (or stress) that you place on your heart. Conditioning your system to slowly and steadily increase the amount of adrenalin it releases to stimulate the heart action is vital to a safe exercise program.

2

With increased heart action, blood circulation increases to deliver more oxygen and nutrients to the working muscles—especially to the legs and arms. As the blood vessels in the muscles dilate and the tendons and ligaments (i.e., connective tissues) are stretched, the muscles become more supple. It is phenomenal to realize that during maximal exercise (which usually occurs during the aerobic phase of your program) the muscles may require as much as 100 times more blood than when at rest![1] The warm-up provides this transitional period between resting and maximal exercise.

3 and 4

Preparing your muscles, tendons, ligaments, and joints for a **safe**, comfortable, more injury-free activity hour is the primary reason that **stretching to increase one's flexibility** is included in the warm-up phase.

Flexibility refers to the **range of motion of a certain joint and its corresponding muscle groups.** To understand how stretching improves range-of-motion in the joints and is vital to your warm-up, visualize your muscles looking like rubberbands. If you continually, slowly lengthen and shorten rubberbands or muscles, each will become **warmer** and more supple after numerous repetitions. For muscles this is because circulation has increased the amount of blood working in the area.

"Cold" muscles and connective tissues are those which have not been given the opportunity to experience an increase in blood, oxygen, or nutrient supply. They are so labeled because no increase in temperature has taken place prior to the intense workout. Cold muscle and connective tissue is less flexible, less ready for a complete range-of-motion usage and, therefore, is more susceptible to muscle and connective tissue injuries like tears and strains.

5

We all desire a comfortable workout session followed by a healthy recovery and over-all feeling of well-being. Many individuals—students and instructors alike—will claim that you must, however, tolerate muscle soreness to have a really effective workout. No pain, no gain is the philosophy. This philosophy is unfounded.

If **static** stretching to warm up the muscle and connective tissues is taught and performed correctly—maintaining the correct positions and quantitatively performing a moderate number of repetitions—you will **not** be sore for the next two days after you begin a conditioning program; and, you will not continually be sore after workouts. It feels good when it's done correctly and does not cause pain[2] (Figure 4-1).

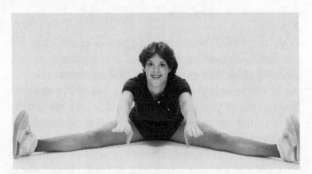

Figure 4-1. Stretching properly does not cause pain.

There are specific techniques enumerated in this chapter on how to stretch properly and if these are followed, stretching will be a pleasurable, mentally relaxing experience.

6

Developing a unique kinesthetic awareness of each muscle group being toned has several advantages. First, if you are able to concentrate on isolating a specific muscle group, stretching and relaxing it during the warm-up (or later the cool-down), you will become more aware of its usage during the aerobics or strength development portions of your workout, or throughout your work and leisure day. Proper usage will enable you to perform work well. Improper usage will result in pains and problems.

Being able to concentrate on stretching and relaxing one muscle group at a time will also give you a background on understanding the voluntary conscious relaxation techniques that come at the conclusion of the workout hour. How to mentally remove tension in a muscle group is a unique skill to acquire. Learning proper stretching technique is the first step in fostering this learning process.

7

And finally, a key benefit derived from the warm-up phase of your program is giving yourself the needed **time** to make the transition of "switching gears," from work to play. Allowing yourself to be totally involved in an exercise workout will provide you with a positive outlet for the stressors in your life!

Caution: If you have had physical injuries and/or recent surgery, particularly of the joints and muscles, or if you have been inactive for a period of time, consult your physician before starting a stretching, strength, or aerobic program.

Improper Stretching Techniques

Before you learn the types of stretching and how to stretch properly, let's clear up the improper, or incorrect, stretching ideas that you may already have in your mind.

1

Your objective is not to concentrate on attaining extreme flexibility. This leads to overstretching and injury.

2

When you stretch too far, you **tighten** the muscles you are trying to stretch! A "stretch reflex" occurs, which means that when a muscle is stretched too far, a nerve reflex responds by sending a signal to the muscles to contract. This, then, keeps the muscles from potential injury.

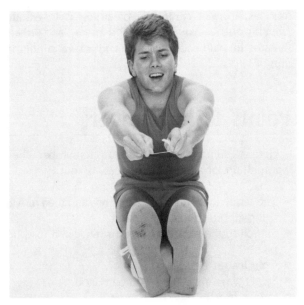

Figure 4-2. Improper stretching will cause pain and physical damage due to microscopic tearing of minute muscle fibers.

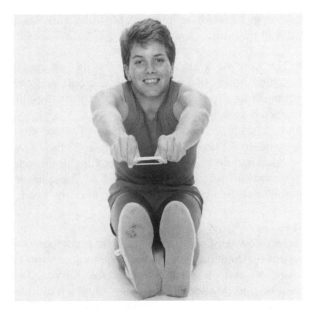

Figure 4-3. Static stretching to "stretch pull."

3
Improper stretching will cause pain and physical damage due to microscopic tearing of minute muscle fibers (Figure 4-2). This leads to the formation of scar tissue in the muscle, with gradual loss of elasticity.[3]

Proper Stretching Techniques

To begin your warm-up stretching prior to an aerobic dance workout, perform **static stretching. Static stretching** is slow, active stretching, with the position held at the joint extremes. You gently stretch the muscle (Figure 4-3) until "stretch pull" (not a pain, but a tight feeling) is reached. You then continue to stretch a little beyond this point, **without motion**, for several seconds. At present, static stretching is considered the most effective method of increasing flexibility.[4] Research has shown that greater gains in flexibility around a specific joint may be made with a training program of static stretching exercises. This type of continuous, long stretching produces greater flexibility with less possibility of injury, probably because it stretches the muscles under controlled conditions.

To end your warm-up phase, **ballistic stretching** can now be included. **Ballistic stretching** (bouncing stretching) is rapid and active, like bobbing and twisting motions. It puts a muscle in a longer-than-resting position by bouncing against the muscle in an attempt to produce greater muscle length. Ballistic stretching can be dangerous if the muscle is cold[5] (i.e., without an increased blood flow present). It can cause a muscle to tighten and could tear it if the muscle has not received adequate blood flow (i.e., "warmed up").

After the static stretching exercises have been performed in the warm-up routine, some ballistic type of warm-up stretching, carefully used, could then be included. These are specifically performed to condition the body for the very quick, dynamic (using space), forward, backward, or lateral movements that you will soon be doing during the aerobic and/or strength training portion of your workout hour.

Remember: A complete routine of static stretching exercises should be included before ballistic stretching exercises are performed, in order to reduce the possibility of injury.

Warm-Up Stretching

Here are a few guidelines to follow to make your stretching warm-up an enjoyable experience:

1
Begin in a sitting position, then stand, and stretch in moving positions (both stationary and through space). Directionality will include lateral, forward, backward, and up and down stretching movements that naturally flow from one to the next.

2
Stretch laterally (to the side) **before** stretching in a forward plane.

3
Stretch with your chin reaching and leading forward

(and eyes forward) as much as possible. This has a twofold purpose:

- The front neck area is one of the first groups to "show aging" of any other muscle group, and any time you can purposefully stretch this normally contracted area, you should.
- A "chin-reach" stretch position will allow your spine to be kept in a straight plane. Excessive "forehead on knee" position stretching to the side or forward will place extra stress on the spine in the neck area because of the weight of the head.

4

Select slow-tempoed (speed) music to accompany the warm-up stretching, and in the beginning perform all exercises at a pace that is comfortable for you. This will help to develop an awareness of which muscles are working and how much improvement is taking place in each succeeding work-out.

Later, if stretching is choreographed to music, it is again performed to a slow-tempoed song. The song should have a 4/4 count (beat). Each stretch position is held for either four or eight counts, according to the kind of stretch performed. You then relax for an equal number of counts (four or eight).

5

The amount of time needed for a complete warm-up varies with the individual, since each person is at a different level of fitness. A general guideline would be a minimum of five to ten minutes of stretching.

6

Discipline yourself to warm up by stretching before every workout, then follow **immediately** with a strenuous rendition of the aerobic dance alphabet or a routine. The stretching benefits dwindle as time passes between warm-up and workout.

7

The **technique** for executing the warm-up stretching efficiently and safely is to **gently ease into a controlled, stretched position and hold it as you gently press.** You push or press to the point of tightness (not pain) so that you feel the muscles working. At the point where you feel the muscles working, mentally relax your mind and "**hold**" a few seconds (approximately four); then slowly physically **relax and withdraw.** Performing the same stretching on the opposite side of your body always follows.

8

Breathe while you exercise. Out-in-out-in. Don't hold your breath and turn red! Breathing properly helps to facilitate the delivery of extra oxygen to the working muscles. Correct controlled breathing is to **exhale** (breathe out) as you **stretch and press;** and **inhale** (breathe in) with each **recovery and relaxation** of the muscle.

Points To Remember

Here is a summary of key points to remember when warming up for an aerobic dance workout:

- The sequential order is to sit, stand, and then move, using all directions throughout.
- Stretch to the side before you stretch in a forward plane.
- Chin lead is best.
- Select slow music to accompany you.
- Stretch at your own pace initially.
- Allow five to ten minutes minimum duration daily.
- Follow **immediately** with the strenuous portion of your program.
- Cues are "stretch," "hold," "relax." Repeat on the opposite side of your body.
- Exhale as you stretch; inhale as you recover.
- Smile and enjoy it! The rewards are soon to come.

A Warm-Up Stretching Routine

The following exercise routine incorporates the previously mentioned goals, guidelines, and techniques. If you are just beginning this program and/or are coming from a previous injury to any muscle group or joint, **begin with care and modify the positions described** as your physician has directed.

Remember: The unique feature of this text is that all exercises are described and photographed by a "mirroring" technique. **You simply perform all of the exercises in this text as you see them shown!** Thus, your **right** side will be the model's actual **left** side, but you perform as directed to the **right.**

Directions

Continue in the **last** position when a new exercise begins, unless noted to change.

To Begin

Sit tall on "sitting" bones, with legs wide-stride and tightly tensed, toes tightly flexed and pointing to the sky, and palms resting on thighs.

Lateral Neck Stretch

1

(Imagine that you are following the flight of a plane taking off, flying high, and then landing.) Look to your extreme right side, eyes **down**.

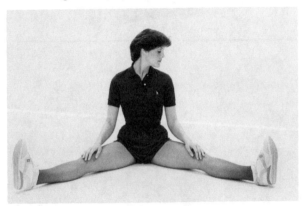

Figure 4-4.

2

Eyes travel **up**ward to the high-right side position. Neck is in a controlled stretch, chin-leading action.

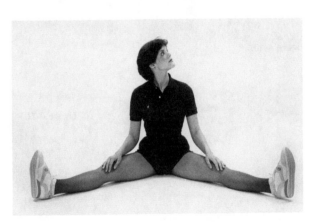

Figure 4-5.

3

Stretch neck **over** to your far left looking high;

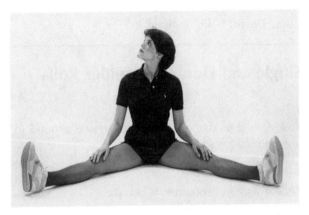

Figure 4-6.

4

. . . then **down** to your far left. **8 counts.**

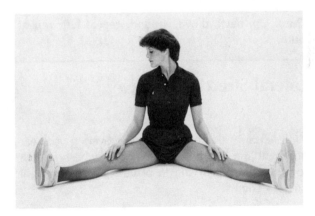

Figure 4-7.

5

Reverse sequence of exercise. **8 counts.**

6

Repeat all. **16 counts.**

Cues: Down, up, over, down.

Shoulder Shrug

1
With eyes forward and thumbs behind knees now, keep same position and stretch and press shoulders **down** as far as possible. **Hold. 4 counts.**

2
Keeping spine erect, lift shoulders **up** to ears. **Hold. 4 counts.**

3
Repeat all, 2 more times. **16 counts.**

Cues: Down, hold, up, hold.

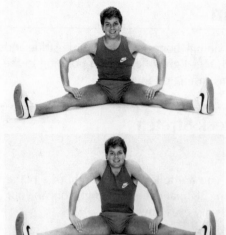

Figure 4-8.

Figure 4-9.

Single and Double Shoulder Rolls

1
Roll right shoulder **up, back, down,** and **around** in one continuous motion. **4 counts.**

2
Repeat with left shoulder. **4 counts.**

3
Simultaneously roll **both** shoulders up, back, down, and around in one continuous motion. **4 counts.**

4
Repeat all 2 times. **24 counts.**

Cues: Up, back, down, around; repeat left; repeat both.

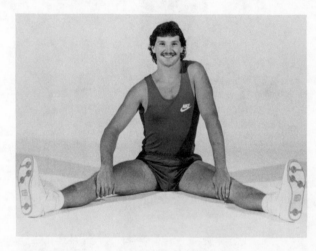

Figure 4-10.

Lateral Stretch 'N Hug

1
With left arm stretching overhead covering your ear and right arm in a hug, pulling across chest, **stretch** toward **right** leg, trying to place right ear on right knee. **4 counts.**

2
Sit tall, arms shoulder high over toes, with toes still slightly flexed skyward. Heels will be slightly off the floor. **4 counts.**

3
Repeat exercise to the **left. 4 counts. Sit tall. 4 counts.**

4
Repeat all one time. **16 counts.**

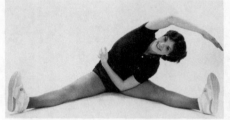

Figure 4-11.

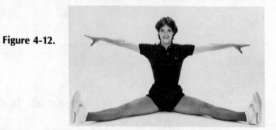

Figure 4-12.

Cues: Stretch right, sit tall, stretch left, sit tall.

Wide-Stride Press

1

Stretch with **chin-lead** over **right** leg, arms parallel and pressing past feet. **8 counts.**

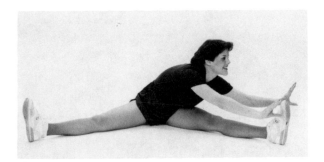

Figure 4-13.

2

Sit tall. 8 counts.

3

Stretch center, with chin-lead, arms parallel and pressing forward. **8 counts.**

4

Sit tall. 8 counts.

3

Advanced only: Grab ankles, chin-lead, eyes forward. Press forward by pulling at ankles. **8 counts. Note:** Any time you press by slowly pulling, it is an **advanced only** stretch. **All other individuals:** Place hands/palms in the vicinity of the ankles and simply **reach. 8 counts.**

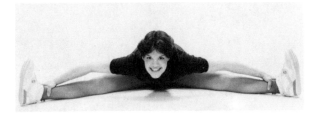

Figure 4-14.

4

Sit tall and recover. **8 counts.**

5

Repeat to the **left** leg; **sit tall; center; sit tall. 32 counts** total.

Cues: Chin-lead right, sit tall, stretch center, sit tall, chin-lead left, sit tall, stretch center, sit tall.

Sandwich Press

1

Slide legs **together,** stretch palms over feet, chin parallel to floor. **8 counts.**

2

Sit tall to recover. **8 counts.**

3

Repeat **forward press. 8 counts.**

4

Sit tall. 8 counts.

Cues: Together and press, sit tall, forward press, sit tall.

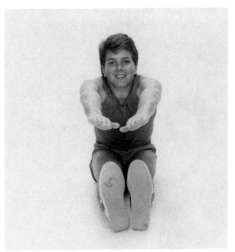

Figure 4-15.

Tailor Sit

1

Draw both feet in toward your center, soles together. Be sure that you are **sitting tall.** Place elbows on thighs, palms over ankles. **4 counts.**

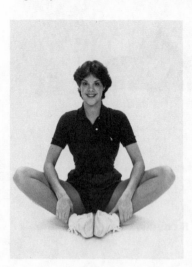

Figure 4-16.

2

Press shoulders and elbows firmly **down. 4 counts.** Knees will come closer to floor.

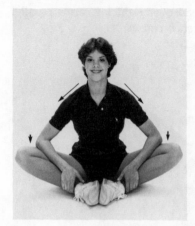

Figure 4-17.

3

Repeat entire exercise once again. **8 counts.**

Note: The more inner leg flexibility you have, the more "flat to the floor" your legs will appear; with less flexibility, the more "froglike," or knees-skyward, your legs will appear. If inflexible, go slowly on this stretch, or you will be sore the next day!

Cues: Sit tall and press down.

Body Wave

1

Raise to a **kneeling** position, with your body erect, arms separate, and shoulder high. Take **4 counts.**

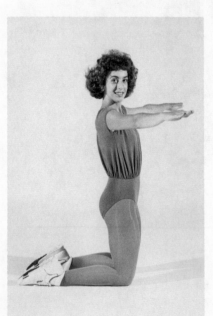

Figure 4-18.

2

Twist trunk to one side, lowering that shoulder and hand. Raise your other shoulder and hand diagonally skyward. Keeping spine firm, **lean** backward **and touch** your heel. **2 counts.**

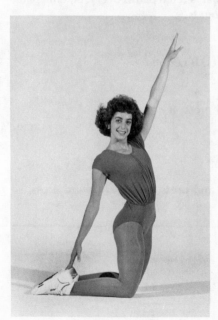

Figure 4-19.

3

Slowly raise, and **twist** trunk to alternate side, lowering that shoulder and hand and raising opposite shoulder and hand diagonally skyward. Repeat **touch. 2 counts.**

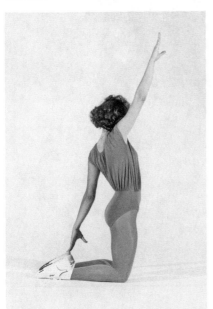

Figure 4-20.

4

Alternate sides 4 times, for **16 counts** total.

5 *Advanced*

Touch the floor behind your foot keeping your body in good position. Slowly raise and repeat to alternate side. **4 counts** per side.

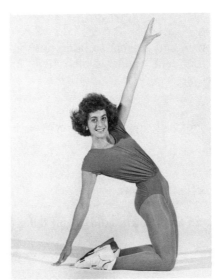

Figure 4-21.

6

Stand now with good posture (taking **16 counts**).

Cues: Raise and kneel, twist-lean and touch, twist-lean and touch; lower; lower (if advanced is also performed). **Stand.**

Lateral Bend 'N Stretch

1

With feet parallel and one foot apart, place left arm up, covering left ear. Leaning to the right, **bend right** hip, lowering right arm down parallel and close to leg. Entire left side—from hip socket to elbow—will be pulled (by gravity on right side) in a tight **stretch. 8 counts.**

2

Stand tall and recover, with arms shoulder high and parallel to floor. **4 counts.**

3

Repeat to **left** side; **stand** tall. **12 counts total.**

Cues: Bend right and stretch; stand; bend left and stretch; stand.

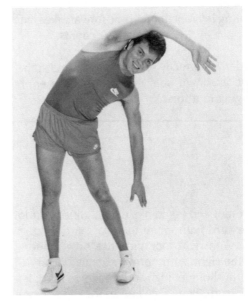

Figure 4-22.

Forward Bend 'N Stretch

1

With feet in same position, bend forward (**bending** knees) and grab ankles on the outside. Slowly lower your head so that the top of your head points to the floor.**8 counts.**

2   *Advanced Only*

Straighten knees now and attempt to bring nose in closer to knees. Do not bounce-stretch here to achieve. **8 counts.**

3

Stand tall, arms stretched skyward, and recover. **8 counts.**

4

Repeat entire exercise. **16 counts.**

Cues: Forward bend and stretch, hold; stand tall.

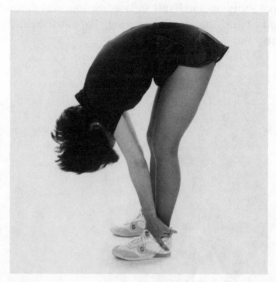

Figure 4-23.

Forward Lunge

1

With feet remaining parallel and **forward** at all times, step two or three feet forward with your right foot. Keep both heels flat on the floor at all times. Place arms forward, parallel and shoulder high, wrists flexed. Keeping spine **erect** and buttocks down, bend right knee only, and as much as you can. **8 counts.**

2

Relax and bring left foot through and forward (keeping right foot in place). Repeat stretch. **8 counts.**

Note: In order to correctly see feet, knees, and spine, this exercise is shown from the side, but the entire body is lunging in a **forward** plane.

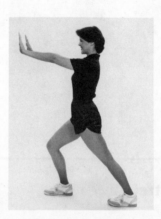

Figure 4-24.

Cues: Lunge forward, hold; walk-through and lunge forward, hold.

Side Lunge

1

Keeping left foot and leg in place (i.e., knee and foot pointing **forward** with entire foot **flat** on the floor), **lunge** right, with right foot and knee **now pointing directly to the right.** Arms form the capital letter "L" (i.e., right arm shoulder high and parallel to floor; left pointing skyward). Bend right knee only, and as much as possible. **Hold. 8 counts.**

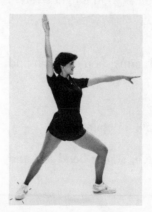

Figure 4-25.

2

Reverse the lunge to the left now by swiveling direction of feet. Right foot now faces forward and left foot points left. Arms are reverse letter "L" or at the nine o'clock position. Bend left knee only and as much as possible. **Hold. 8 counts.**

Cues: Lunge side, hold; reverse and lunge side, hold.

Knee Lift

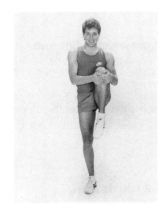

Figure 4-26.

1

Shifting weight to center, turn left foot forward and take weight on it. **Lift** and encircle right knee and bring knee **to** your chest, keeping your spine tightly erect. **Pull** knee closer to chest and hold, with standing leg locked. **8 counts.**

2

Reverse and repeat with left knee. **8 counts.**

Cues: Lift and pull, hold; repeat left lift and pull, hold.

Quad Stretch

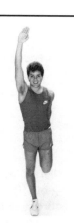

Figure 4-27.

1

Drop right knee down, pointing to the floor, and **grasp** your right ankle with your right hand (behind you). Raise left arm skyward. With legs **together, pull** right leg until knees line up side by side. Be sure to maintain pelvis in tucked position, abdomen in, chest high. **8 counts.**

2

Repeat with left knee. **8 counts.**

Cues: Grasp and pull, hold; repeat left—grasp and pull, hold.

Ankle Stretch

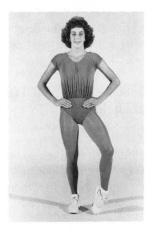 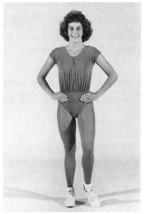

1

Stand with weight on left foot, hands on hips, and feet slightly apart. Rotate right foot **outward** making 4 circles. **8 counts.**

2

Rotate right foot **inward** making 4 circles. **8 counts.**

3

Repeat with left foot **outward** and **inward**, 4 circles each. **16 counts.**

Cues: Circle out, circle in; reverse and circle out, circle in.

Figure 4-28.　　　　　**Figure 4-29.**

Note: Ballistic—Bounce and Stretch begins with these last exercises to conclude the warm-up stretching.

Twisting Toe Touch

1
Stretch skyward, with feet one foot apart. **1 count.**

2
Twist entire body to **right**, from knees to fingertips. **1 count.**

3
Bend at the waist and **touch** fingertips to the floor beside your right shoe or as close as you can get to it. **2 counts.**

4
Stand again, **turn forward. 2 counts total.**

5
Repeat entire sequence to **left (6 counts total),** finishing with full standing stretch.

Cues: Stretch skyward, twist right, bend and touch, stand, turn forward; repeat left.

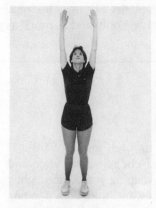
Figure 4-30.

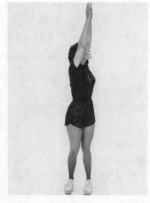
Figure 4-31.

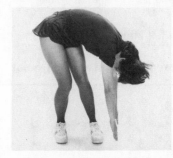
Figure 4-32.

Arm Circles

1
Stretch arms out at sides, shoulder height, with **wrists** tightly **flexed,** fingers spread facing out. Rotate arms in **small** to medium **circles** using **entire** stretched arm. Repeat 8 times **backward,** slowly. **16 counts.**

Cues: Wrists flexed and circle small, 2, 3, 4, 5, 6, 7, 8.

2
Perform **large backward** arm **circles,** palms facing down, with heels **lifting** when hands are at the height of the circle and heels **lowering** when arms are lowered. **2 counts.** Repeat 4 times. **8 counts.**

Cues: Circle large palms-in-blades back and lift, lower; lift, lower; lift, lower; lift, lower.

3
Relax and lower arms to shoulder height, palms down and continue backward, but now with **small** low arm circles. Feet begin a **side** step right, **touch** left; then **side** step left, **touch** right. **4 counts.**

Cues: Lower and small circles, and side, touch, side, touch.

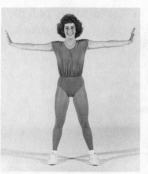
Figure 4-33.

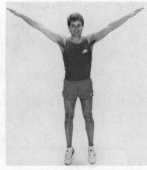
Figure 4-34.

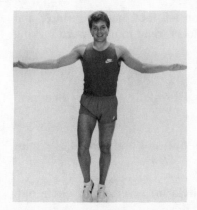
Figure 4-35.

Adding Variety to Your Stretching Program

Having a partner, using various sports equipment (ropes, weights, balls, etc.), or having the entire group exercise in contact with one another can add variety to your stretching program. Be creative and develop more ideas of your own (or do it as a class project and enjoy the creative ideas of many other people).

A Reminder: The exercises used for warm-ups can also be used for cool-downs by just reversing the order. You begin from a slow walking, to a sitting, and finally to a lying down position for the cool-down.

Bridging the Activity Between Stretching and Aerobic Dance: The Warm-Up Jog or Rope-Jumping Phase

To complete the warm-up phase and condition the legs for the impact movement to come, try jogging or jumping rope for the duration of one medium-tempoed song. Begin with a shorter two-and-one-half-minute jog, or jumping rope, and condition until you can later eventually last for a complete five-minute fast-tempoed song. This conditioning will also give you two more aerobic-type activities from which to choose, for your aerobic fitness program.

Beginner Programs

If you fitness-tested to be "very poor," "poor," or "fair," jog or jump rope using the following progression. It will gradually build your endurance and skill in each activity:

Try intervals of one-half minute of jogging or jumping rope followed by one-half minute of walking. Increase the aerobic jogging or jumping rope by one-half-minute intervals as you are able, still providing the recovery walking one-half-minute intervals in between. Your goal is to last for a two-and-one-half-minute to five-minute song, without the recovery-walk interval. This will conclude your warm-up program phase.

Advanced Programs

If you tested in "good," "excellent," or "superior" fitness condition, jog or jump rope **continuously** for the duration of one medium-tempoed song.

If jumping rope, try to jump, first, **every other beat** for the entire song. This will help you to develop your basic skill of jumping rope. Condition your legs to reach a goal of jumping the rope for **every beat** of a fast-tempoed five-minute song.

More Details on Jogging and Rope Jumping

Proper **jogging** technique includes having the foot contact the floor in a **heel first** position, outer half of the foot second, and push-off from the great toe area last. Arms are loosely held bent at sides, with hands held in loose fists. Opposite arm and leg are in a forward position.

For **jumping rope** you need a rope of correct length, and preferably a giving surface upon which to jump. The correct length of rope is for it to reach your armpits when held down tightly under your feet with a few extra inches, or a handle, with which to hold the rope comfortably. If no handles are present, tape the ends or tie knots in the ends of sash cord to help prevent fraying.

Figure 4-36.

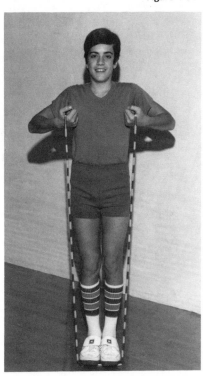

Try a variety of rope jumping skills:

1

One foot and then the other. If you jump on only one foot, do no more than four repetitions on the same foot. Alternate immediately to the other foot for the same number of reps.

2

Two feet at a time.

3

Jump **crossed**, followed by a one-foot or two-foot jump.

4

Hopscotch jump, i.e., two-foot jump stride, one-foot jump, two-foot jump stride, alternate one-foot jump (shown below).

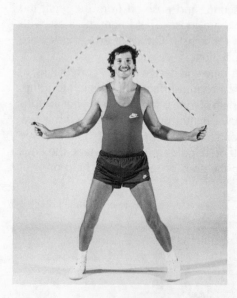

Figure 4-37.

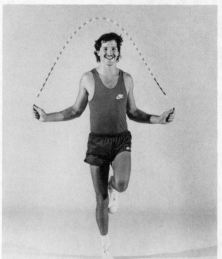

Figure 4-38.

Summary

The warm-up portion of your workout hour is the vitally important transitional phase between a rather inactive resting state of the body and mind, to one that is safely ready for the twenty to thirty minutes of intense aerobic dance next to come!

The following is an index review of all of the warm-up exercises which were presented in this chapter, in **sequential-routine** order:

- Lateral Neck Stretch
- Shoulder Shrug
- Single and Double Shoulder Rolls
- Lateral Stretch 'N Hug
- Wide-Stride Press
- Sandwich Press
- Tailor Sit
- Body Wave
- Lateral Bend 'N Stretch
- Forward Bend 'N Stretch
- Forward Lunge
- Side Lunge
- Knee Lift
- Quad Stretch
- Ankle Stretch
- Twisting Toe Touch
- Arm Circles—
  - Small, Wrists Flexed
  - Large, Backward with Heel Lifts
  - Small and Low, with Side and Touch Steps
- Warm-Up Jogging Technique
- Warm-Up Jumping Rope Varieties—
  - One-Foot Jump
  - Two-Foot Jump
  - Crossed, followed with One/Two-Foot Jump
  - Hopscotch Jump

5

THE ABC'S OF
AEROBIC DANCE

The aerobic dance phase of the workout is a series of gesture and step patterns put to music and performed in a continuous, rhythmical way. Once the dance phase of the program is begun, stay on your feet and keep moving through all aspects of the workout (dancing, walking, pulse taking, etc.). The workout should continue for a minimum of twenty minutes in order to exercise the heart muscle enough to reach your goal of achieving the training effect (Chapter 1). (**Note:** It may take several workouts of shorter duration for you to become conditioned enough to reach the twenty-minute minimum.)

Pacing Yourself

Learning to pace yourself during the workout is imperative for you to reach and stay within your training zone. It may be necessary in the beginning to "walk through" (doing the steps without bounce or tension) the basic skills and then gradually increase the intensity. As you practice and learn the aerobic dance A-B-C's possibilities, your body will become conditioned to the point where you will be able to bounce, hop, and jump more, use greater amounts of muscle tension, lift the knees higher, and get more height in your kicks with less effort.

Pacing can be disrupted by gesture and step patterns that you find difficult. To alleviate this situation, individualize your program by creatively changing the difficult gesture and/or step patterns into movements that are easier for you to master.

Learning Your ABC's. . .

Here are a few suggestions to help you to learn the alphabetized gesture and step patterns that follow:

1
Learn one gesture or step pattern at a time. Repeat it several times until it is mastered.

2
Count out the beats as you perform each step/gesture pattern with medium-tempoed music. (Music has a steady beat that is called a count. A beat or count is the unit that measures time. The steady count is the underlying beat to the melody or song.)

3
When a gesture or step pattern is mastered, learn either another item in that alphabetized listing, **or** proceed on to the next letter category of the alphabet. In this way, at the conclusion of your course/program, you will end up with a working knowledge of **at least one** aerobic dance possibility from each alphabetized category. Spontaneous and creative improvisation will follow!

4
If you select to learn—consecutively—all of the patterns in one alphabetical category presented here, **review them immediately after learning that alphabetical letter**, by performing each for **four repetitions**, one after another. Concentrate on the transition

from one step pattern to the next. This will develop your ability to combine various patterns, in order to be able to plan (choreograph) your own dances in several weeks!

5

If a pattern seems difficult to perform, start by walking through it slowly, performing first the step pattern, then the gestures (always maintaining arms at, or above, waist level), and finally combining them together. When the entire pattern is mastered, **then** increase the pace to an "aerobic" intensity.

6

Be sure the music you select to initially learn the patterns is of a slow or medium tempo. Save the fast-tempoed music for your learned choreographed combinations when you can add muscle tension, bounce, hops, and jumps for an increased heart-rate intensity.

7

If you are aerobically fit (i.e., can pass a fitness test as described in Chapter 1) **and you understand and have established good position (exercising postures) for aerobic dance movement**, consider the following alternative to your regular workout program. Try the step and gesture patterns holding or wearing **one-to-three-pound hand or wrist weights**, to not only encourage muscle definition in your arms and upper torso, but also to speed up caloric energy expenditure. You'll need to compensate for the force that the weights will exhibit by performing **more controlled, slower movements** so that injury does not occur.

PRECAUTION: It is imperative to be physically fit—aerobically—BEFORE you add weights to your workout, during the AEROBIC portion of your hour.

You want to be sure your heart and lungs are ready for the increased workload, before the goals of increased muscle-definition or faster fat-weight-loss is begun, during the **aerobic** portion of your hour.

8

In order to keep frustration down to a minimum, just remember that this is not "performance dance," it is recreational-fitness dance and technique perfection is not necessary. It is only important that you **keep moving** so that your main goal of aerobic capacity improvement is realized. And in regards to technique, you will note that the fingers are spread in many of the pictures. This gesture, called **jazz hands** (Figure 5-1) stretches the hand and forearm muscles, keeping tension throughout the upper body too, and not just in the legs and feet.

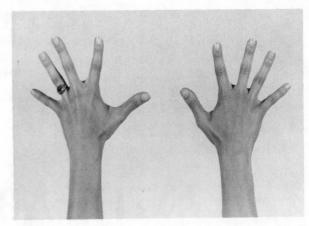

Figure 5-1.

9

Because every individual learns at a different pace, or, may come into a program with various limitations (either temporary like reduced ability from a cold, or from a chronic problem like a prior knee injury), it is important to continually individualize your program (correctly adapting the movements) so that you are able to **safely** perform them.

10

Finally, perhaps the most important suggestion to never forget, is to thoroughly **enjoy** rhythmically moving aerobically to music. So smile! Having patience with yourself in class to methodically learn the various possibilities, and then practicing the patterns during your own workout time at home, is an excellent training habit to establish. With a little effort, this activity can prove to be a great source for the relief and management of stress in your life, whether in class or at home.

Catalogue of Aerobic Dance Gesture and Step Patterns

The following selections are only the beginning of possible gesture and step patterns appropriate to this fitness activity. Dance step or pattern **cues** are in boldface type. **Weight-bearing foot**, or important movement, **is accented with slash marks throughout the text.** Also, all exercises are photographed and described by the "mirroring technique" (described in the Preface).

At the conclusion of the descriptions, an alphabetized list of all the gesture and step patterns presented in the chapter is given. This list will prove to be an invaluable source for both review and for planning your own choreographed dances (as detailed in Chapter 8).

In addition, this list includes **cues** for each gesture and step pattern described here, for quick reference and easy recall.

"A-B-C-D"
(A Bounce-Coordination Dance Pattern)

Note: This pattern can be performed rhythmically to any 4/4 time music, as follows, or in any improvised way. There are three basic directional positions and one "hold" position. This can be performed in one repetition as described here, or it can be performed as an **entire** aerobic dance as described next.

1
Bounce on left foot, with right foot **forward**—toe pointed and tapping. Arms are stretched **forward**, parallel, and thumbs down. **1 count.**

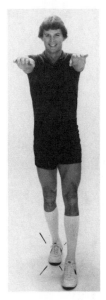

Figure 5-2.   Figure 5-3.

2
Bounce (again) on left foot, with right foot out to right **side** (toe pointed and tapping). Arms are shoulder high and out from **sides**, thumbs down. **1 count.**

3
Bounce (again) on left foot, with right foot **back** behind you (toe pointed and tapping). Fingers are stretched—wide **back** behind your head, elbows out. **1 count.**

4
Bounce and **hold** on both feet **together.** Arms are

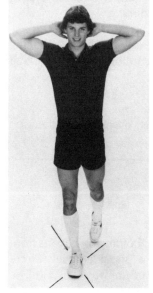 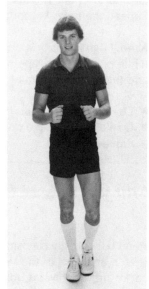

Figure 5-4.   Figure 5-5.

close to the body, elbows down at sides, with hands in jogging position. **1 count.**

5-8
Reverse and repeat bouncing on right foot, tapping left foot **forward, side, back, together,** moving arms in the same gestures as described in **1-4. 4 counts.**

"A-B-C-D" Aerobic Dance

Suggested Sequence of These Movements:

1
Repeat four times, right foot pointing and tapping **each** direction (i.e., **forward** 4, **side** 4, **back** 4, **hold** 4). Repeat four times, left foot pointing and tapping (bouncing on right).

2
Repeat three times, right foot pointing, but **before each directional change,** shift weight on **both** feet together, with arms close to body, one time (i.e., a **hold and bounce** once would be the fourth count for a 4/4 time rhythm). **Forward** 3/**hold** 1/**side** 3/**hold** 1, **back** 3/**hold** 1, **hold and bounce** 4). Repeat three times, left foot pointing.

3
Repeat two times, right foot pointing.
Repeat two times, left foot pointing.

4
Repeat one time, right foot pointing (each direction; the fourth count is **shift** 'n hold, two feet in place).
Repeat one time, left foot pointing.

Note: High intensity is to do as listed above (bouncing while pointing and tapping). To lower your work load and thus your heart rate:

- Don't bounce but do both arms and legs.
- Don't bounce and lower or eliminate the arm moves.

- Don't do the leg movements, just arm movements, especially with 1- to 5-pound hand weights.
- And, for an extremely high-intensity, high-impact conditioning workout, add a **HOP** instead of **bounce** throughout. Be sure to alter the sequences, however, so you are only **one-foot-hopping on the same foot not more than 4 consecutive times** (i.e., 4 right forward, 4 left forward, 4 right side, 4 left side, etc.).

This bounce-coordination rhythmical dance can thus be as much, or as little, exercise that each participant can (aerobically) do. For variety, have the entire group form a large circle, facing in, and perform the exercise as a group!

Arm Circle

1
Stand tall with good posture, holding body parts firm. Stretch arms out to the side at shoulder level. **Circle** backward, downward, forward, upward quickly. The emphasis is on the backward motion. **1 count or 2 counts.**

Cues: Circle-back.

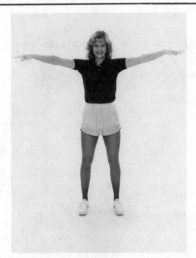

Figure 5-6.

Bounce, Two Feet

1
In place with arms extended to the side at shoulder level, **lift** to the balls of both feet and **lower**.

Note: If this is done quickly it takes **1 count. Cue: Bounce.** If this is done slower it takes **2 counts. Cues: Lift, bounce.**

2
For variety, separate feet forward and backward and use push-pull **punching** arms as you **bounce. 1 or 2 counts.**

Cues: Punch, bounce.

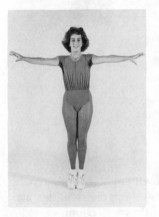

Figure 5-7.

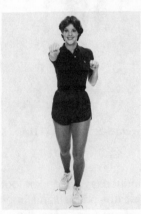

Figure 5-8.

Bounce-Step, Bounce-Touch

1

The right arm extends forward at shoulder level as the left arm extends left. Bounce-**step** on the right foot. **1 count.**

2

In the same position, **bounce and touch** the left foot forward with the leg extending. **1 count.**

3

Reverse the step. The left arm extends forward at shoulder level as the right arm extends right. **Bounce-step** on the left foot. **1 count.**

4

In the same position, **bounce and touch** the right foot backward, with leg extended. **1 count.**

Cues: Bounce-step, bounce-touch; bounce-step, bounce-touch.

Bounce Steps, With Side-Touch

1

Two-foot **bounce** in place. **1 count.**

2

One-foot bounce on right foot while left foot extends sideward to left and **touches. 1 count.**

3

Draw left back in close and two-foot **bounce. 1 count.**

4

One-foot bounce on left foot while right foot extends sideward to right and **touches. 1 count.**

Cues: Bounce, touch, bounce, touch.

Cha-Cha

Begin with weight evenly balanced.

1

Cross left foot over right, *taking weight on the left foot.* **1 count.**

2

Step right foot **back** and to right side. **1 count.**

3

Step left foot to left side quickly. ½ **count.**

Step right foot to right side quickly. ½ **count.**

4

Step left foot to left side. **1 count.**

5-8

Reverse and repeat to opposite direction. **Cross** right over left (*taking weight with right*), step left **back** and to left, **step** right quickly, **step** left quickly, **step** right. **4 counts.**

Cues: Cross, back, step-step, step; cross, back, step-step, step.

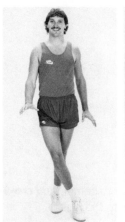
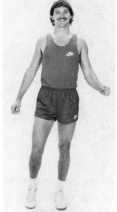
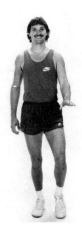
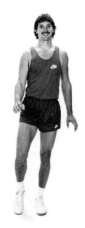
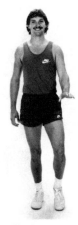

Figure 5-9.   Figure 5-10.   Figure 5-11.   Figure 5-12.   Figure 5-13.

Cha-Cha, With Kick Pattern

1
Cross right foot over left foot. **1 count.**

2
Step **back** on left foot. **1 count.**

3
Step right to right side. **1 count.**

4
Keeping weight on right foot, **kick** left leg forward. **1 count.**

5
Step left. **1 count.**

6
Step right. **1 count.**

7
Step left quickly. **½ count. Step** right quickly. **½ count.**

8
Step left. **1 count.**

Repeat using the same feet in same direction. **8 counts.**

Cues: Cross, back, step, kick, step, step, step-step, step.

Charleston Flapper Walk

1
Step right, **swinging** both arms to the right side of the body, elbows bent, fingers spread wide. **1 count.**

2
Bend the right knee as the left knee **lifts** up and the arms **swing down** in front. **1 count.**

3
Reverse **1 and 2**, stepping on the left foot. **2 counts.**

Cues: Step and swing, lift and swing down; left and swing, lift and swing down.

Cross-Step Forward, Touch To The Side

1
Cross-step forward on the right foot, bending both knees. Arms are shoulder level, hands touching, elbows bent. **1 count.**

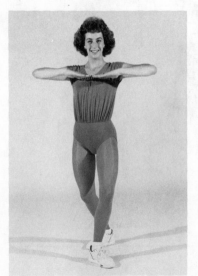

Figure 5-14.

2
Touch the left foot to the left side with leg extended.

Turn the head to the left and extend the arms to the side at shoulder level. The right foot is bearing the weight. **1 count.**

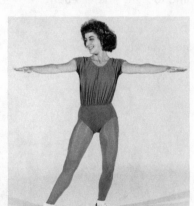

Figure 5-15.

3
Reverse by bringing arms back in to center, and **cross-stepping** forward on the left foot. **1 count.**

4
Touch the right foot to the right side, leg extended. Turn head to right side as arms are extended sideward. **1 count.**

Cues: Cross, touch; cross, touch.

Cross-Step, Hop

1

With weight evenly distributed, step on the right foot with the knee bent, **crossing** in front of the left foot. Arms are extended to the side at shoulder level. **1 count.**

2

Holding **1** position, **hop** on the right foot. **1 count.**

3

Reverse **1 and 2**, **cross-stepping and hopping** with left foot. **2 counts.**

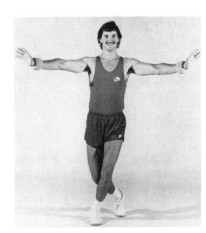

Figure 5-16.

Cues: Cross, hop; cross, hop.

Doubles: Knees and Kicks

1

Step left and **lift** right knee up, touch it **down** to the floor, lift it **up**, touch it **down**. Hands slap raised knee, or clap. **4 counts.**

Cues: Knee-lift, down, up, down.

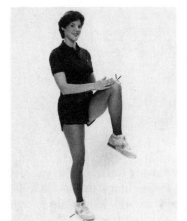

Figure 5-17.

2

Weight remaining left, **kick** right leg up, touch it **down** to the floor, kick it **up**, touch it **down**. Bring arms up to shoulder level for the kicks. **4 counts.**

Cues: Kick, down, up, down.

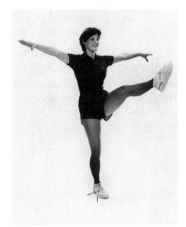

Figure 5-18.

Double Hops

1

Hop on the right foot, lifting the left knee and holding the arms at the waist, hands making fists. **1 count.**

2

Hop on the right foot with the left knee lifted and the right arm **punching** downward. **1 count.**

3

Reverse **1 and 2**, hopping on the left foot and punching with left arm. **2 counts.**

Cues: Hop, hop and punch; hop, hop and punch.

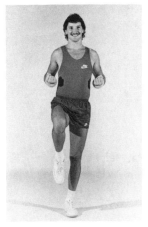

Figure 5-19.

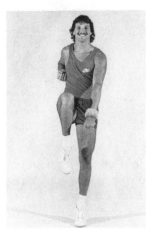

Figure 5-20.

Double Hop, Hitch Kick

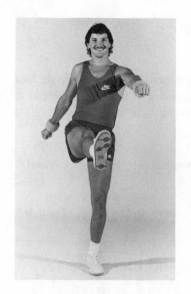

1

Hop on the right foot, bending and lifting the left knee. Arms are drawn in near sides with fists facing forward. **1 count.**

2

Hop on the right foot, **kicking** the left leg forward. The right arm extends forward as you punch with your fist. The left arm extends to the back. **1 count.**

3

Reverse **1 and 2**, **hopping** on the left foot, and **kicking** the right leg. **2 counts.**

Cues: Hop, hop-kick; hop, hop-kick.

Elbow-Wipers

1

Lunge to the left side with your right foot forward in the lunge. **Hold** three counts. **4 counts.**

2

Place left palm on top of your head, elbow **pointing** in the direction of the lunge and head facing front-away from the lunge. Right hand is held stationary on the right hip throughout the pattern. **Hold. 2 counts.**

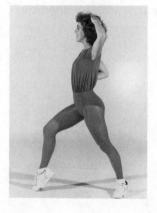

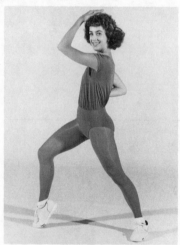
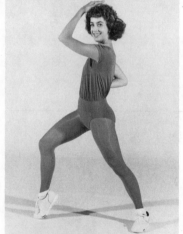

Figure 5-22.

3

Hold lunging leg position, rotate left elbow **wide** open to your side as you rotate your head toward the lunge. **Hold. 2 counts.**

4

Repeat elbow and head gestures **2 and 3. 4 counts.**

5

Reverse and repeat by walking through with your left foot (it's now forward in the **lunge** to the left side). **Hold** lunge three counts as you switch arms, right palm now on top of head, left hand at left waist. **4 counts.**

6

Point right elbow toward the lunge, head facing toward the back. **Hold. 2 counts.**

7

Rotate right elbow **wide** open pointing to the back, as head faces the lunge. **Hold. 2 counts.**

8

Repeat elbow and head gestures **6 and 7. 4 counts.**

Cues: Lunge and hold, two, three, four, point, hold, wide, hold, point, hold, wide, hold; walk-through and lunge, (hold) two, three, four, point, hold, wide, hold, point, hold, wide, hold.

Fall Back 'N Jump Forward Pattern

1

Facing front, **step** with the **right** foot to the right side. Arms extended to the side at shoulder level throughout the entire pattern. **1 count.**

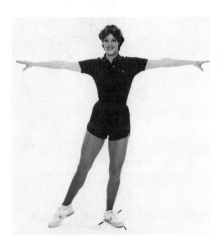

Figure 5-24.

2

Quickly **step** with the **left** foot next to the right foot, and **step** with the **right** foot quickly to the right side. **1 count.**

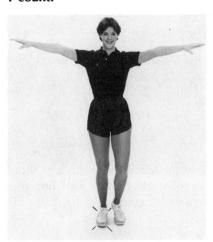

Figure 5-25.

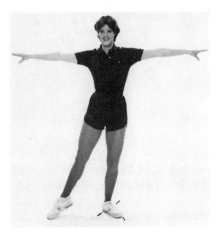

Figure 5-26.

3

Traveling to the right side, turn the body diagonally left as you jump **back** on the left foot, kicking the right leg forward (diagonally left). **1 count.**

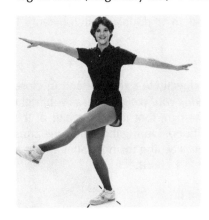

Figure 5-27.

4

Still facing diagonally left, jump **forward** on the right foot, kicking the left leg backward, knee bent. **1 count.**

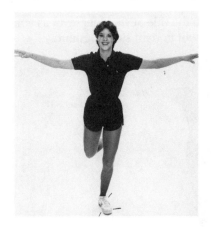

Figure 5-28.

5

Reverse entire pattern. Facing front, **step** with the **left** foot to the left side. **1 count.**

6

Quickly step with the **right** foot next to the left foot, and step quickly with the **left** foot to the left side. **1 count.**

7

Traveling to the left side, turn the body diagonally right as you jump **back** on the right foot, kicking the left leg forward (diagonally right). **1 count.**

8

Still facing diagonally right, jump forward on the left foot, kicking the right leg backward, knee bent. **1 count.**

Cues: Step, step-step, back, forward.

Gallop

1

Step right foot to right side. Arms and hands are held parallel, down, and in a double "hitch-hiker." **1 count.**

2

Slide your left foot directly to right side and in close to your right foot *taking your weight on it* as your right knee bends and **lifts** right foot up to the ball of the foot (but not off the floor). During the slides, the arms are raised waist-high, keeping them parallel and in a double "hitch-hiker." **1 count.**

Cues: Step, slide and lift.

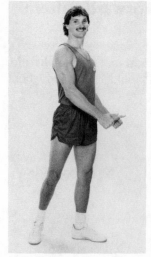
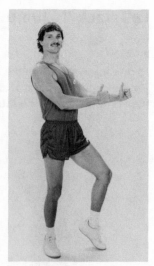

Figure 5-29.   Figure 5-30.

Grapevine

1

Arms straight, out to the side at shoulder level as you step with the right foot to right **side. 1 count.**

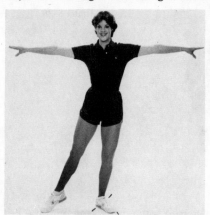

Figure 5-31.

2

Step with the left foot **back** behind the right foot. **1 count.**

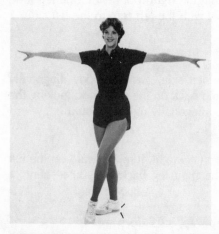

Figure 5-32.

3

Step with the right foot to the right **side. 1 count.**

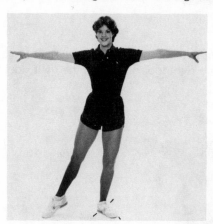

Figure 5-33.

4

Bring left toe in close and **touch**, with arms kept shoulder high, but now bent at elbows, with fingertips touching, thumbs down. **1 count.**

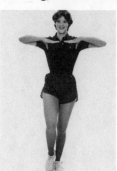

Figure 5-34.

Reverse and repeat *1, 2, 3, 4* by: Step **side** left, step **back** right, step **side** left, **touch** right. **4 counts.**

Cues: Side, back, side, touch; side, back, side, touch.

Grapevine, Varieties

Instead of **touch** as the fourth step with elbows bent, try one of these variations:

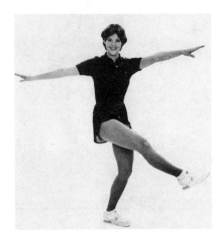

Figure 5-35.
Grapevine 'n
Kick

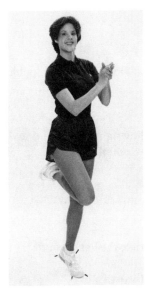

Figure 5-36
Grapevine 'n Hop

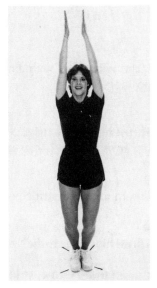

Figure 5-37.
Grapevine 'n Jump-Clap

Heel Out, Toe In Hop Pattern

1
Hop right, with left heel **out** forward. **1 count.**

2
Hop right, with left toe **in**, near other foot. **1 count.**

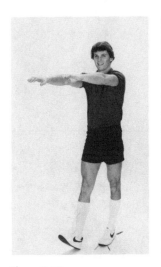

Figure 5-38.

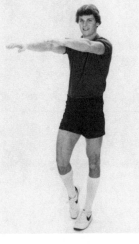

Figure 5-39.

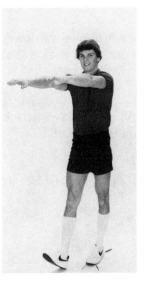

Figure 5-40.

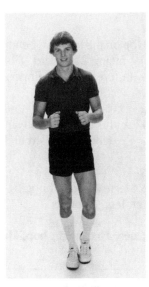

Figure 5-41.

3
Hop right, with left heel **out** forward. **1 count.**

4
Two-foot **jump** together, with weight transferring, then, onto left foot to repeat; arms in close, jogging position. **1 count.**

5-8
Reverse and repeat hopping left with right heel out, in, out, two-foot jump.

Cues: Out, in, out, jump; out, in, out, jump.

Hip Thrust

1

Stand **widestride** with arms at sides in loose jogging position. **1 count.**

2

Thrust hips to the right, bending right knee and drawing arms directly backward. **1 count.**

3

Return to center **stride** position *1.* **1 count.**

4

Thrust hips again to the right; or to the left. **1 count.**

Cues: Stride, thrust; stride, thrust.

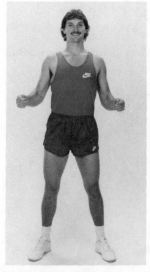 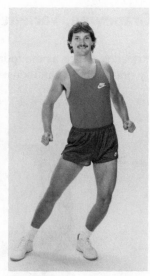

Figure 5-42.   **Figure 5-43.**

Hop, Kick

1

Hop on the left foot, bending the right knee with lower leg facing backward. Elbows are down at the sides, with forearms and fingers skyward. **1 count.**

2

Kick the right leg forward and through arms which are extended forward and parallel. **1 count.**

3-4

Reverse *1 and 2,* hopping on the right foot and kicking left leg. **2 counts.**

Cues: Hop, kick; hop, kick.

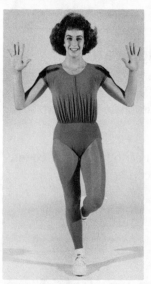 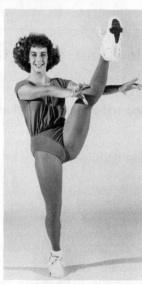

Figure 5-44.   **Figure 5-45.**

Hopscotch

1

Jump to a **widestride** position with knees bent, landing on the balls of both feet. Arms are extended to the side at shoulder level. **1 count.**

2

Hop forward on the right foot, bringing the left foot behind the right knee (bending the left knee). Be sure that the right foot is brought under the body for better balance. **1 count.**

3

Repeat *1,* jump to **stride. 1 count.**

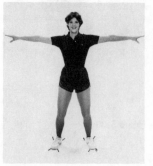 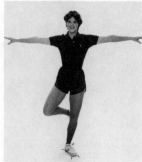

Figure 5-46.   **Figure 5-47.**

4

Reverse *2* by **hopping** forward on the left foot. **1 count.**

Cues: Stride, hop; stride, hop.

Hopscotch, Variety

2 and 4

For variety, touch hand down and behind to the raised foot, while raising other arm diagonally skyward. **1 count.**

Cues: Stride, hop-touch; stride, hop-touch.

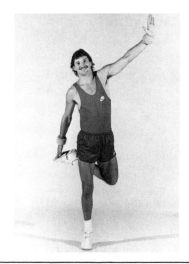

Figure 5-48.

Hustle

Traveling forward:

1
Jog right.

2
Jog left.

3
Jog right.

4
Lift the left knee as you hop on the right foot and **clap. 4 counts.**

5-8
Traveling backward:
Jog back left, **jog** right, **jog** left and **lift** right knee as you hop on left foot and **clap. 4 counts.**

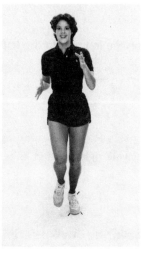 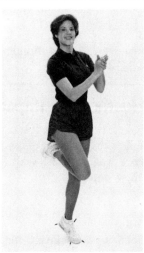

Figure 5-49.   Figure 5-50.

Cues: Jog, jog, jog, lift-clap; jog back, jog, jog, lift-clap.

Hustle, Cross-Elbow Touch

1
Jog three times, starting with the right foot, arms in jogger's position. **3 counts.**

2
Hop on the right foot, lifting the left knee up. At the same time, **touch** the left knee with the right **elbow. 1 count.**

3
Reverse **1 and 2**, starting on the left foot and then touching left elbow to right knee. **4 counts.**

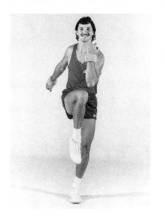

Figure 5-51.

Cues: Jog, jog, jog, elbow-touch; jog, jog, jog, elbow-touch.

Hustle, High-Impact Variety

1
Facing front, **hop** on the right foot to the right side, holding the arms at the waist, hands making fists. **1 count.**

2
Hop on the left foot next to the right foot. **1 count.**

3
Hop on the right foot to the right side. **1 count.**

4
Hop on the right foot as the left knee **lifts** up. The right arm punches down. **1 count.**

5
Reverse **1, 2, 3, 4,** hopping on the left foot to the left side. **4 counts.**

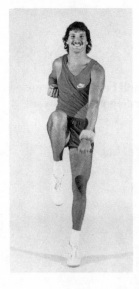

Figure 5-52.

Cues: Hop, hop, hop, lift; hop, hop, hop, lift.

Hustle, Low-Impact

1-4
Pace walk forward, **walk** left, **walk** right, **lift** left knee up. **4 counts.**

5-8
Pace walk backward left, **walk** right, **walk** left, **lift** right knee up. **4 counts.**

Cues: Walk, walk, walk, lift; walk, walk, walk, lift.

Note: You can enjoy a low-impact movement like this and still receive the benefits of a high-intensity workout by using **weights** held in the hands (1 to 5 pounds).

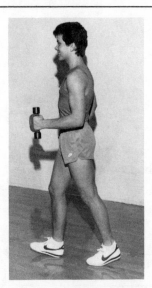

Figure 5-53.

Itchy Strut

1
With arms at your sides, grasping your thighs throughout pattern, **step** right foot forward. **1 count.**

2
Lift left shoulder and knee, open and to the left side. **1 count.**

3
Step left foot forward. **1 count.**

4
Lift right shoulder and knee, open and to the right side. **1 count.**

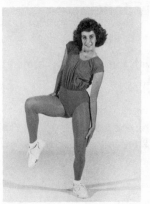
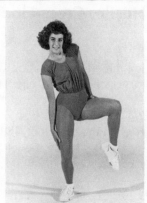

Figure 5-54.   Figure 5-55.

Cues: Step, lift; step, lift.

Jazz Touch-Out 'N In Pattern

1

With weight kept on right foot, stretch left leg **out** to left side. Arms are kept shoulder high and stretched to out position also. **1 count.**

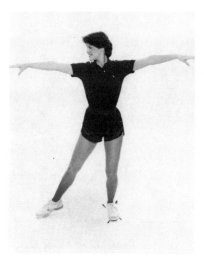

Figure 5-56.

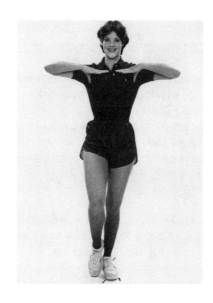

Figure 5-57.

2

Bring left toe **in** close and touch, with arms kept shoulder high, but now bent at elbows, with fingertips touching, thumbs down. **1 count.**

3

Repeat, **out. 1 count.**

4

Instead of left just touching, you **shift** and take **your weight** now on left. **1 count.**

5-8

Repeat entire pattern in reverse, with weight on left. (You end with weight shifted to right.) **4 counts.**

Cues: Out, in, out, shift-your-weight; out, in, out, weight-right.

Now continue right on with this next pattern—

Jazz Touch—Forward 'N Backward pattern

1

With weight kept on right, stretch left leg **forward** and touch. Opposite arm (right) stretched forward, same arm (left) stretched backward. **1 count.**

2

Swing arms to their opposite extremes while swinging left leg **back** and touching. (Keep weight on right.) **1 count.**

3

Repeat, **forward. 1 count.**

4

Instead of left just touching, you **shift** and take your **weight** now on to left. **1 count.**

5-8

Repeat entire pattern in reverse, beginning with right

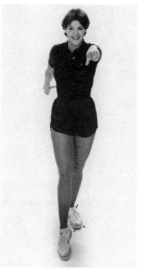

Figure 5-58.

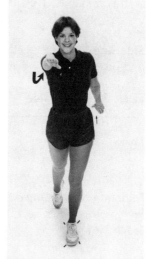

Figure 5-59.

leg stretched forward (and left arm forward). For high intensity, add **hop** between touches. **4 counts.**

Cues: Forward, back, forward, shift-your-weight; forward, back, forward, weight-right.

Jazz-Walk

1

Start with weight evenly balanced, facing forward. Right fist is on right hip, with left arm in a straight-down position in front of your body.

With weight on your left foot, **touch-side wide** to the right side with your right foot. **Swing** your left arm up chest high and wide open to the left side with elbow bent **and click** left fingers. **2 counts.**

2

Step on the right foot (taking weight on it now). **Swing** left arm across chest, **clicking** fingers as you **cross-side-touch** left foot to the right side. **2 counts.**

Cues: Touch-side-wide, swing-click; step, swing-click and cross-touch.

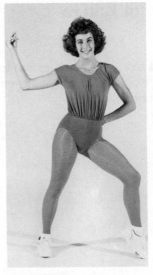
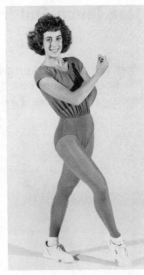

Figure 5-60.   Figure 5-61.

Jazz Side-Walk

Begin with head down, arms directly down in front of you with fingers stretched wide in jazz-hands position.

1

With weight on your left foot, **step-wide** to the right **side.** Head turns to look low and left as left arm extends and right arm flexes—both pointing directionally left with jazz-hands. **1 count.**

2

Side-step left foot **together,** close to right foot, arms and head maintaining the same gestures. **1 count.**

Cues: Step-side-wide, together.

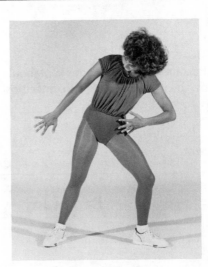

Figure 5-62.

Jog

1

Facing front, start **jog** on the right foot. Arms at waist level with elbows bent, hands in loose fists. **1 count (each jog).**

Note: Proper jogging technique is foot contacting the floor **heel-first,** outer half of the foot second, with push-off on the ball of the foot last.

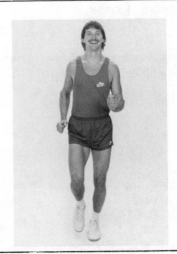

Figure 5-63.

Jog Circling

Cues: Jog, two, three, four, five, six, seven, eight.

1
Jog eight times starting with the right foot. Starting to your right side, continue traveling in a circle. End facing front on the eighth jog. **8 counts.**

2
Repeat to your left side, traveling in a circle. **8 counts.**

One-Foot Jump

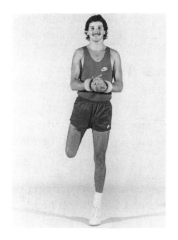

Figure 5-64.

1
Jump upward, taking off with the **right** foot as the left foot kicks backward with a bent knee. Elbows are bent close to the sides and hands clap. **1 count.**

2
Alternate and **jump** upward, taking off with the **left** foot as the right foot kicks backward with a bent knee. **1 count.**

Cues: Jump-right; jump-left.

Two-Foot Jump

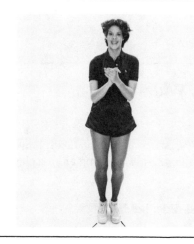

Figure 5-65.

1
In place, **jump** upward, taking off with the balls of both feet. Land on the balls of both feet, flexing the ankles, knees, and hips, and **clap. 1 count, or 2 counts.**

Cues: Jump-clap! (1 count) Jump and clap! (2 counts).

Circling Jumps

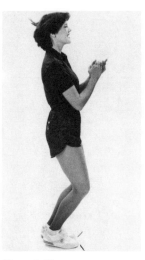 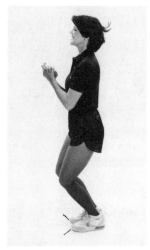

1
Begin with feet together and facing forward. Moving clockwise, jump and clap using a two-foot jump, to the right side—**3 o'clock. 1 count/2 counts.**

2
Jump and clap to the back side—**6 o'clock. 1 count/2 counts.**

3
Jump and clap to the left side—**9 o'clock. 1 count/2 counts.**

Figure 5-66.   Figure 5-67.

4
Jump and clap forward, as shown in the Two-Foot Jump—**noon. 1 count/2 counts.**
5-8
Reverse and repeat circling jumps moving counterclockwise: jump and clap **9 o'clock, 6 o'clock; 3 o'clock, midnight. 4 counts/8 counts.**

Note: 1 count each if jump-clap are done simultaneously; **2 counts** each if jump and clap are done separately.

Cues for 1 count each: 3 o'clock, 6 o'clock, 9 o'clock, noon; Reverse-and-9 o'clock, 6 o'clock, 3 o'clock, midnight.

Cues for 2 counts each: add a **hold and clap** after each direction.

Forward 'N Backward Jumping

1
Take off from both feet, jump **forward**, landing on both feet with arms extended above the head. **1 count.**

2
Take off from both feet, jump **backward**, landing on both feet, with arms extended above the head. **1 count.**

Cues: Jump forward, jump back.

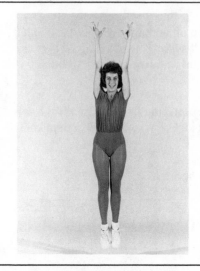

Figure 5-68.

Jump 'N Land, Widestride

1
Extending arms in a "V" shape above the head, **jump** into a **widestride** position. **Hold,** keeping all muscles firm. **2 counts.**

Cues: Jump and land-wide, hold.

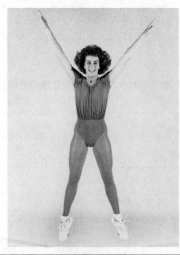

Figure 5-69.

Side Jump, Clap

1
Jump widestride to the right **side**, bending the knees. **1 count.**

2
Clap your hands to the right side. **1 count.**

3
Reverse *1* **and** *2*, jumping and clapping to your left. **2 counts.**

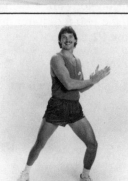

Figure 5-70.

Cues: Jump-side, clap; side, clap.

Ski Jump

1

Place left upper arm and elbow against the left side of the body, extending left forearm out away from the left side, with hand in a fist facing upward. Extend right arm diagonally right and skyward with hand in a fist facing downward. With feet together, two-foot **jump** to the right **side. Hold. 2 counts.**

2

Reverse arm gestures and repeat two-foot **jump** to the left **side. Hold. 2 counts.**

Cues: Jump-side, hold; jump-side, hold.

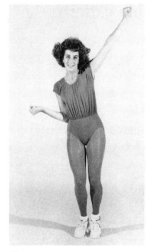
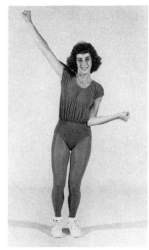

Figure 5-71.   Figure 5-72.

Jumping Jacks, Regular

1

Jump to **stride, clapping** hands above your head. **1 count.**

2

Two-foot jump feet in close **together,** as you bring arms down to sides, hands **slapping** thighs. **1 count.**

Cues: Stride-clap, together-slap.

Note: When performing jumping jacks within a choreographed dance, repeat steps **1 through 2** for two or four repetitions.

If performing as a high-intensity and impact conditioning program perform steps **1 through 2** for 8 to 10 repetitions. Follow with a low-impact activity interval for 8 to 10 counts (like walking in place, etc.). Continue these intervals until you become winded, **taking note of the number of jumping jack repetitions and sets you perform** (i.e., jumping jacks 10 times, repeating 3 sets, for a total of 30 jumping jacks). Then, work up to one-continual-minute intervals of jumping jacks, with half-minute walking around your space.

Crazy Jumping Jack

1

Jump and land on both feet in a wide**stride** position. Arms are extended to the side at shoulder level; knees are flexed. **1 count.**

2

Jump, **cross**ing the right foot in front of the left, while crossing arms above your head. **1 count.**

3

Repeat **1, stride. 1 count.**

4

Repeat **2, cross**ing the right foot in back of the left. **1 count.**

Cues: Stride, cross; stride, cross.

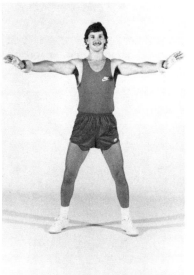
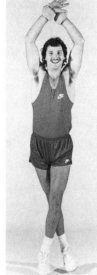

Figure 5-73.   Figure 5-74.

Jumping Jacks—Double Pattern

1
Jump to wide stride, arms wide; cue by **"letter X"**. **1 count.**

2
Jump to legs together, arms high and together clapping; cue by **"letter high I"**. **1 count.**

3
Jump to wide stride, arms wide; cue by **"letter X"**. **1 count.**

4
Jump to legs together, arms down at sides; cue by **"letter low I"**. **1 count.**

Cues: X, high I, X, low I.

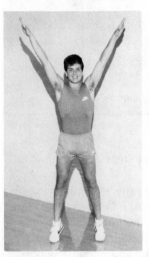
Figure 5-75.

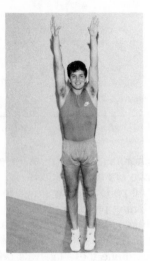
Figure 5-76.

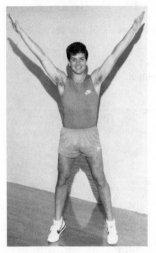
Figure 5-77.

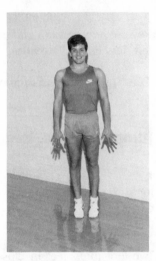
Figure 5-78.

Knee-Lift, Varieties

1-2
Step and **knee-lift** (the other leg) to a waist-high position. **Touch elbow** to raised knee in one of the following variations. **2 counts.**

Cues: Step-lift, elbow-touch (-same, -open, or -crossed); repeat left.

SAME
Knee-elbow touch forward on the **same** side, first lift right; then left. **4 counts.**

OPEN TO SIDE
Knee-elbow touch **open** wide to the right side; then to the left side. **4 counts.**

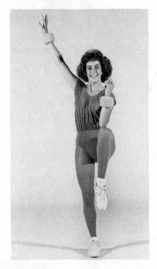
Figure 5-79.

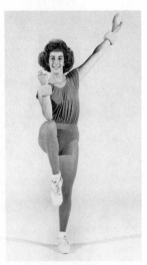
Figure 5-80.

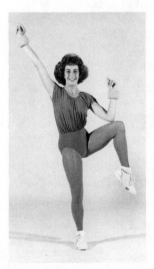
Figure 5-81.

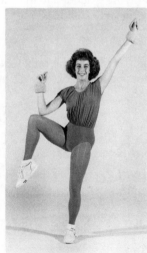
Figure 5-82.

CROSSED

Knee-elbow touch **crossed,** with the right knee to left elbow; then left knee to right elbow. **4 counts.**

Note: Add a **hop** to any of these variations to increase intensity.

Cues: Hop-lift, elbow-touch-(same/open/crossed).

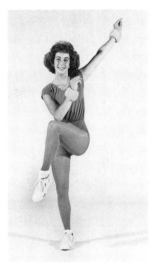

Figure 5-83.

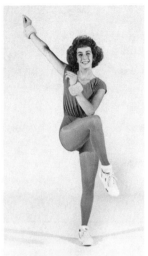

Figure 5-84.

Lunge, Forward

1

Take your weight on your left foot which is turned sideward. With arms forward and parallel and fingers stretched, stretch your entire body far forward and step **-lunge-** on the right foot, which is pointed forward. Your right lunging knee fully bends, with your left leg remaining stretched behind you, and the left foot remaining entirely **flat** on the floor. Body weight is controlled by the strong thigh muscles, with buttocks tucked in a down-and-under position, keeping the spine firm and stabilized.

Take a full eight counts to reach the position, press and stretch, hold, and return to a standing position by taking weight on the forward foot and walking through with the back stretched leg. The backward leg that walks through can immediately **lunge** forward again or take weight to assume a new step pattern. **8 counts.**

Cues: Forward-lunge, 2, 3, 4, 5, 6, 7, 8; walk-through-and-lunge, 2, 3, 4, 5, 6, 7, 8.

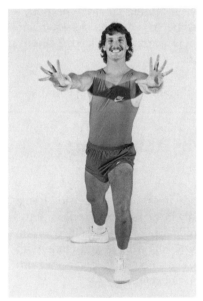

Figure 5-85.

Scissor Lunge

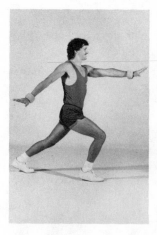

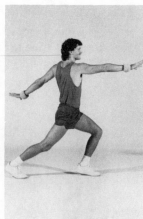

1

Jump forward on the right foot, bending the right knee as the left leg is kept extended back. The left arm is extended forward at shoulder level, and the right arm is extended backward with jazz-hands for emphasis. **1 count.**

2

Reverse **1**, **(scissor) jumping** forward on the left foot. Bend the left knee as the right leg is extended back. The right arm is extended forward at shoulder level and the left arm is stretched back, both with jazz-hands. **1 count.**

Cues: Jump-forward, scissor-jump.

Figure 5-86.   **Figure 5-87.**

Lunge, Side

1

Take weight on your right foot pointing forward. Facing forward with arms shoulder high, extended to the sides, **lunge** left with left foot pointing toward left side wall. The lunging thigh muscle controls the body's sideward lean. Remember to keep buttocks down and under, keeping the spine firm and stabilized. **2 counts, 4 counts, or 8 counts.**

Cues: Lunge-side and count (the holding counts).

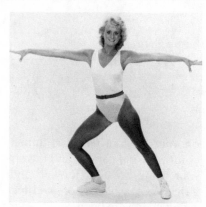

Figure 5-88.

Lunge, Side With Arm Circling

1

Assume the same body position as in the side lunge but now turn head only in the lunging direction. Press the lunging arm, shoulder high and directly over the lunging knee, while making a large arm circle with the back arm. Take eight counts to circle the arm clockwise or counter-clockwise.

Cues: (Arms) 3 o'clock, hold; 6 o'clock, hold; 9 o'clock, hold; noon, hold. Counter-clockwise cues would be the reverse order of these. 8 counts.

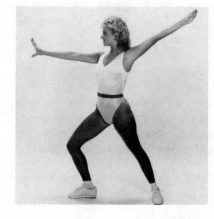

Figure 5-89.

Lunge Side-Bounce 'N Sway

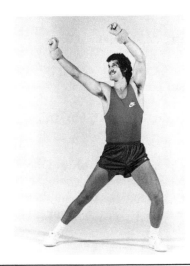

Figure 5-90

1
Raise arms overhead, parallel and diagonally high left as you step and **bounce-lunge** right. **2 counts.**

2
Reverse by shifting weight, swaying and **bounce-lunging** left, swinging arms from the diagonally high left to the diagonally high right position. Your head follows the direction of the arms. **2 counts.**

Cues: Lunge-side and bounce; sway-lunge and bounce.

March

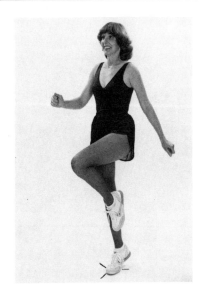

Figure 5-91

1
Marching is a step-lift, one count each, step pattern, and cues are usually given to coincide with the foot contacting the floor, i.e., **left, right** or the direction of the movement, **forward, rear, side,** etc.

—Knees are raised up, parallel to floor with toes always pointed.

—Arms should be swung so that each arm is up when the knee of the opposite leg is up (i.e., left arm is up when right knee is up).

—Think good posture all the time; i.e., "heads up" "shoulders back."**1 count.**

Monkey-Jump Pattern

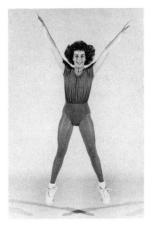 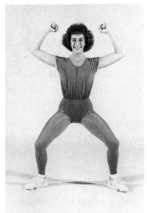

1
Jump with legs in **wide**stride position and arms extended in wide-"V" position. **1 count.**

2
Land facing **forward** in a widestride, bent-knee position. Arms are flexed to the sides (forearms facing up as shown, or down), keeping elbows shoulder high and hands in fists.**1 count.**

3
Maintaining body position in step **2** for the remainder of the pattern, monkey-jump to the **right** side. **1 count.**

Figure 5-92   **Figure 5-93**

4
Monkey-jump to the **back** side. **1 count.**

5

Monkey-jump to the **left** side. **1 count.**

6

Monkey-jump to **forward** position. **1 count.**

Cues: Jump! Forward, right, back, left, forward.

7-12

Reverse direction by first repeating the **forward** monkey-jump, then **left, back, right, forward,** ending with a push-off and up into a wide**stride**, "V"-arm **jump!** Land with feet together, arms at sides. **6 counts.**

Note: This is a fun-jump that is more exciting with "uhh!" sound-effects when landing in each direction!

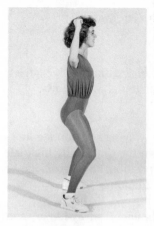
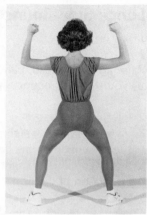

Figure 5-94   **Figure 5-95**

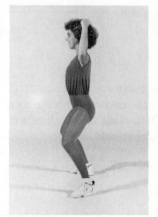
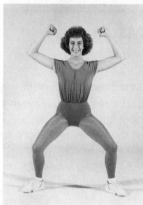

Figure 5-96   **Figure 5-97**

Nasty! Strut

1

Walk into a right **lunge, bending** both knees. **1 count.**

2

With hands in tight fists, **flex** right elbow with forearm up, tightly contracting the bicep muscle. Extend left arm down and back with elbow slightly flexed, tightly contracting upper arm muscles. **Bounce. 1 count.**

3-4

Reverse and repeat by walking (nasty!) into a **lunge** to the left side, **bending** both knees as you reverse your arm gestures. **Bounce. 2 counts.**

Cues: Lunge and bend, bounce and flex; lunge and bend, bounce and flex.

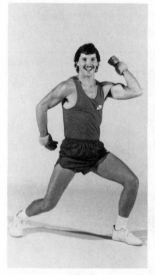
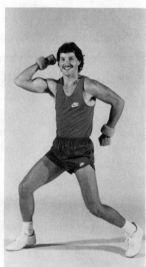

Figure 5-98   **Figure 5-99**

Opposite Punch 'N Point

1
Place right arm at right side throughout. **Step far** right with right foot and bend right knee. **Punch** left arm directly right at shoulder height. **1 count.**

2
Keeping weight on right foot, **swing** left leg forward to the right side, extending leg and foot in a toe-**touch,** as left arm travels across the chest and **punches** back and left at shoulder height. Head follows left arm in a tilt-left. **1 count.**

Cues: Step far and punch, swing-touch and punch.

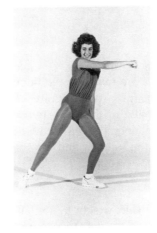
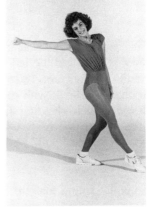

Figure 5-100   Figure 5-101

Polka

1
Hop right, lifting left leg backward and keeping arms out shoulder high. **½ count.**

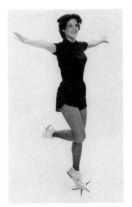

Figure 5-102

2
Step left, in close quickly. **½ count.**

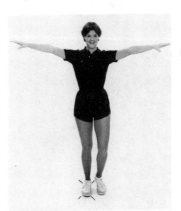

Figure 5-103

3
Step right, in close quickly. **½ count.**

4
Step left, in close quickly. **½ count.**

Cues: Hop-step, step-step.

Reverse **1, 2, 3, and 4** and repeat. **2 counts.**

Polka, Varieites

. . . Circling

Cues: To the right, back, side, forward.

. . . Low-Impact

Cues: Step, step, step, hold; step, step, step, hold.

. . . Side-To-Side

Cues: To-the-left; to-the-right.

Prance

1

Face forward with weight on the right foot. The left knee is bent and the left toes are **touch**ing the floor next to the right foot. The right arm is extended forward at shoulder level with the palm of the hand (wrist flexed)—**push**—leading the action. The left elbow is bent next to the body with the forearm and fingers pointing up in "pull" position. **1 count.**

2

Continue facing forward and **shift** weight to the left foot with the right knee bent and the right toes **touch**ing and arms push-**pull** opposite *1*. **1 count.**

Cues: Touch-push, shift-touch and pull.

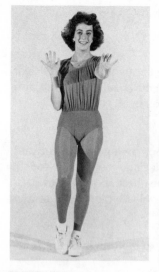
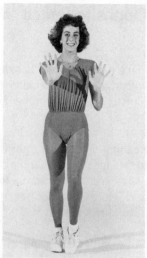

Figure 5-104   **Figure 5-105**

Quads 'N Hams Coordination Pattern

1

Step right; arms shoulder high. **1 count.**

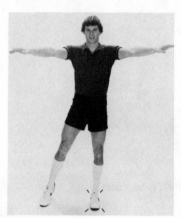

Figure 5-106

2

Lift left foot **forward,** with a toe touch with right hand. Opposite hand and arm high (left). **1 count.**

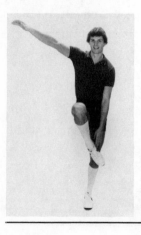

Figure 5-107

3

Step left, arms shoulder high. **1 count.**

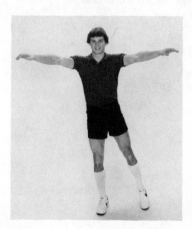

Figure 5-108

4

Lift right foot **backward,** with a toe touch with left hand. Opposite hand and arm high (right). **1 count.**

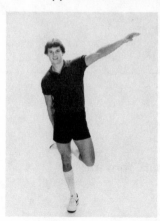

Figure 5-109

Cues: Step, lift-front, step, lift-back.

Reach

1

Step on the right foot to the right side and stretch the entire body to the right side in a wide shape, **reaching** high diagonally right with the right arm. Left hand grasps at left waist while left leg stretches wide and high to the left side. **2 counts.**

2

Reverse and stretch to the other side. **2 counts.**

Cues: Step, reach; step, reach.

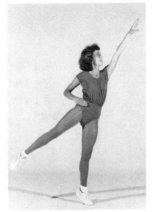 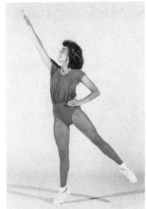

Figure 5-110   **Figure 5-111**

Rock Big, Forward 'N Backward

Note: With all rocking, the body maintains a firm leaning posture, not a collapsing lean forward, backward, or side to side.

1

With arms shoulder high and out to the sides, jump to a **forward** right foot, leaning forward. **1 count.**

2

Rock and lean **backward,** taking weight on left foot, leaving forward foot forward but off the ground. **1 count.**

Cues: Rock-forward and back.

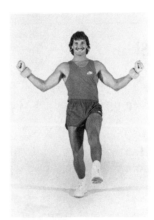

Figure 5-112   **Figure 5-113**

Rock Side-To-Side

1

With arms extended to the side at shoulder level, hop on the right foot to the right **side,** placing weight over the right leg (knee and ankle flexed) as you lift the left leg out to the side. **1 count.**

2

With arms extended to the side at shoulder level, hop on the left foot to the left **side,** placing weight over left leg (knee and ankle flexed) as you lift the right leg out to the side. **1 count.**

Cues: Rock-side; side.

For variety, punch fists and arms sideward in the same direction as the rock.

Cues: Rock-side and punch; side and punch.

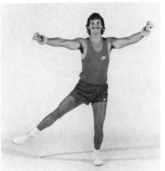

Figure 5-114

Figure 5-115

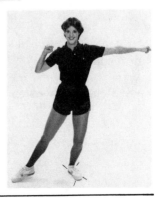

Shake Up, Shake Down

1

In a widestride position, raise to the ball of right foot while extending left arm forward, holding right arm in close to the body, fingers spread. **Shake** your arms, hands, and hips side-to-side four times. **4 counts.**

2

Keeping a widestride position, lean the body forward, extending the arms down. **Shake** shoulders, arms, hands, and hips up and down four times. **4 counts.**

Cues: Shake, two, three, four; shake-down, six, seven, eight.

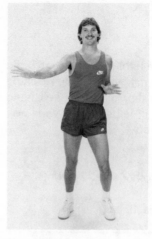 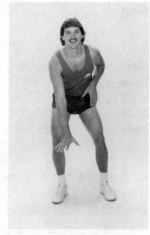

Figure 5-116   **Figure 5-117**

Skip

1

Step right forward. **1 count.**

2

Hop right, lifting left knee forward and upward. **1 count.**

3-4

Reverse and repeat **step, hopping** on left foot. **2 counts.**

Cues: Step, hop; step, hop.

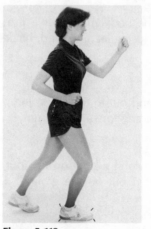 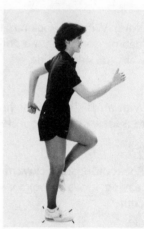

Figure 5-118   **Figure 5-119**

Slides

1

Step right foot directly to right side, reaching with foot as far as you can. **1 count.**

2

Bring feet **together** in mid-air but still moving directly to right. Land and **step** momentarily on left foot. **1 count.**

3

Repeat in repetitions of two or four slides to each side. **4 or 8 counts.**

Cues: Step, together-step.

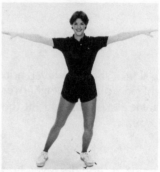

Figure 5-120

Figure 5-121

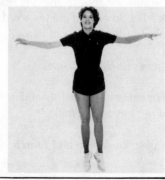

Slide, Bend, Jump, Clap Pattern

1
Step with the right foot to the right side, bringing the left foot next to the right—"**slide**". **1 count.**

2
Bend at the ankles, knees, and hips, as you push your chest out, extend arms up and out to the sides, while tossing head backward. **1 count.**

3
Reach the arms skyward as you **jump** upward. **1 count.**

4
Land on the balls of the feet, flexing the ankles, knees, and hips. **Clap** the hands as you land. **1 count.**

5-8
Repeat to the opposite direction.

Cues: Slide, bend, jump, clap; slide, bend, jump, clap.

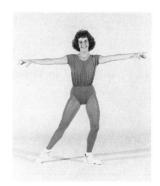

Figure 5-122

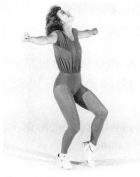

Figure 5-123

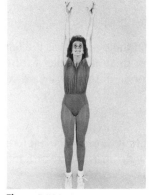

Figure 5-124

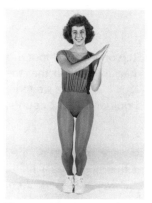

Figure 5-125

"Snob Strut"

1
Side-step forward with left foot as you **touch** right toe wide, side, and forward. Twist trunk and face forward. Extend arms down and out to the sides with palms flat and wrists tightly flexed. **1 count.**

2
Rotate trunk and head facing the back, raising your nose and chin ("**snob**") skyward and **bounce. 1 count.**

3-4
Reverse direction and repeat with the weight on your right foot, and **touch**ing left toe wide, side and forward. Twist trunk and face forward. **Bounce.** Rotate trunk back, "**snob**" gesture, and **bounce. 2 counts.**

Cues: Side-step and touch, "snob" and bounce; twist and touch, "snob" and bounce.

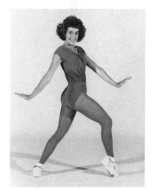

Figure 5-126

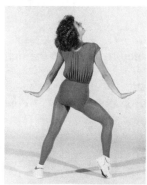

Figure 5-127

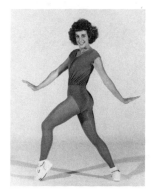

Figure 5-128

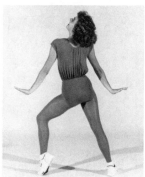

Figure 5-129

Step, Hop

1

Step with the right foot in place, arms held in fists in jogging position. **1 count.**

2

Hop with the right foot in place, lifting the left knee. **1 count.**

Create a variety of arm gesture possibilities!

Cues: Step, hop.

Step, Hop Circling

1

Step on the right foot, **hop** on the right foot as the left knee is lifted so that the left thigh is parallel to the floor. Arms are stretched forward and backward at shoulder level. **2 counts.**

2

Reverse and **step** on the left foot, **hop** on the left foot as the right knee is lifted. Swing arms to forward and backward position. **2 counts.**

3

Step right, **hop** right. **2 counts.**

4

Step left, **hop** left. **2 counts.**

All four of these step, hops are performed circling, one time.

Cues: Step, hop to the side; step, hop to the back; step, hop to the side; step, hop front.

Step, Hop, Step, Kick Pattern

1

Step right foot to the right side. **1 count.**

2

Hop on right foot. **1 count.**

3

Step back on the left foot. **1 count.**

4

Keeping weight on the left foot, **kick** right leg forward. **1 count.**

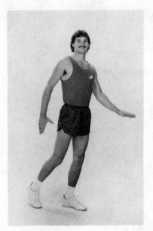 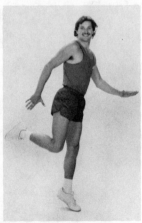 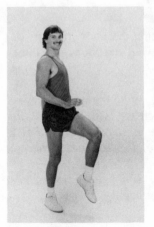 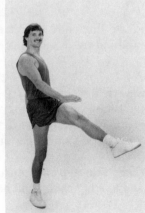

Figure 5-130   **Figure 5-131**   **Figure 5-132**   **Figure 5-133**

Cues: Step, hop, step, kick.

Step, Kick

1
Step on the right foot, bending the left knee. Elbows are bent next to side, forearms and fingers pointing up. **1 count.**

2
Hop on the right foot as the left leg **kicks** forward with the arms extending forward, fingers stretched wide. **1 count.**

3
Reverse and repeat, **stepping** left and **kicking** right. **2 counts.**

Cues: Step, kick; step, kick.

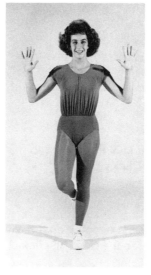
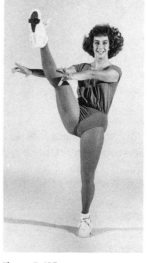

Figure 5-134   **Figure 5-135**

Step, Kick Circling

1
Facing forward, **step** right. Raise arms forward, parallel, and shoulder height and **kick** left foot between arms, to a comfortable height for you. **2 counts.**

2
Now complete a circle, continuing counter-clockwise to the left stepping on the left foot and kicking with the right foot. Continue alternating right foot, left foot, a total of eight times for **16 counts.**

Cues: Step, kick; two; three; four; five; six; seven; eight.

Step, Kick 'N Punch-Down

1
Step right foot to right side. **1 count.**

2
Kick left leg directly to left side as you **punch down** both fists directly in front of you. **1 count.**

3
Raise arms forward, together and up overhead as you **step** on left foot in place. **1 count.**

4
Keeping weight on left foot, **kick** right leg forward as you again lower arms together and **punch down** both fists directly in front of you. Kicking leg is between punching arms. **1 count.**

Cues: Step, kick-side and punch down, step, kick-front and punch down.

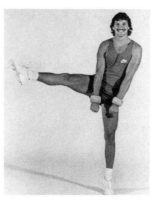

Figure 5-136

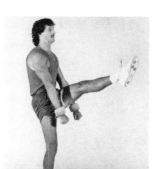

Figure 5-137

Step, Side-Kick

1
Step with the right foot in place, stretching the right arm above the shoulder and the left arm down. **1 count.**

2
Hop on the right foot as you **kick** the left leg to the **side** to a comfortable height. **Click** your fingers as you kick. **1 count.**

3
Reverse **1 and 2** by **step**ping and hopping on the left foot and **kick**ing the right leg to the **side** and **click**. **2 counts.**

Cues: Step, side-kick and click; step, side-kick and click.

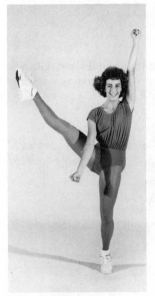 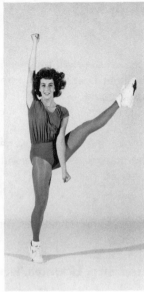

Figure 5-138   **Figure 5-139**

Step, Lift, Touch, Lift Pattern

1
Turn diagonally right and **step** with the right foot to the right side. Arms are extended to the side at shoulder level. **1 count.**

2
Lift the left knee to the right, diagonally. **1 count.**

3
Touch the left foot on the floor diagonally right in front of the right foot. **1 count.**

4
Lift the left knee to the right, diagonally. **1 count.**

5-8
Reverse **1, 2, 3, 4,** starting with the left foot to the left side. **4 counts.**

Cues: Step, lift, touch, lift; step, lift, touch, lift.

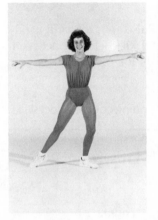 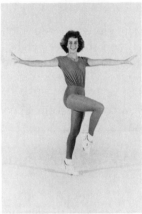

Figure 5-140   **Figure 5-141**

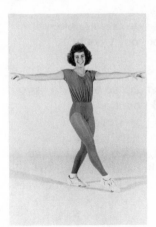 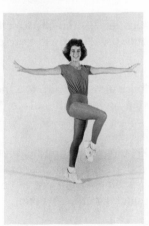

Figure 5-142   **Figure 5-143**

Stride 'N Twist Pattern

1
Jump to wide **stride,** arms shoulder high. **1 count.**

2
Jump to right over left, legs in a **crossed** position. **1 count.**

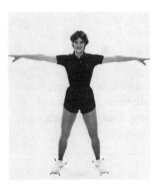

Figure 5-144

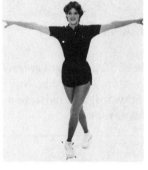

Figure 5-145

3
Turn counterclockwise (or left) on pivoting balls of both feet. **1 count.**

4
"Hold" position **1 count.**

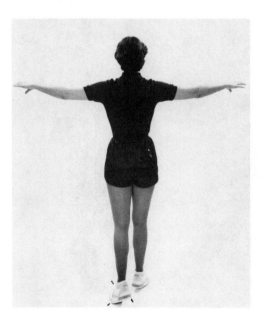

Figure 5-146

5
With weight on left foot, **lift** right knee and touch with palms. **1 count.**

6
Touch right toe down to floor momentarily (not shown here). **1 count.**

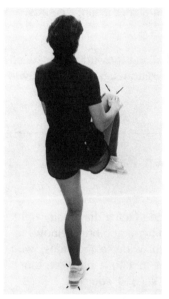

Figure 5-147

7
Kick, diagonally right, through forward stretched arms. **1 count.**

8
Lower kick and **touch** right to floor. **1 count.**

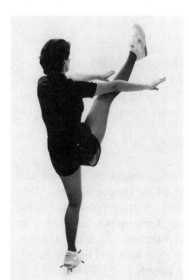

Figure 5-148

Cues: Stride, cross, turn, hold, lift, touch, kick, touch.

The Twist

1

Twist by stepping forward with one foot, and **lowering** entire trunk by a bending of the knees. Keep pelvis tucked under so that spine is erect. Arms are in jogging position, swinging forward and backward as you lower. **4 counts.**

2

Twist again, raising **up** to full stance again. **4 counts.**

3-4

Reverse and repeat by walking forward or backward directly into the twist position again. **Twist-down, twist-up. 8 counts.**

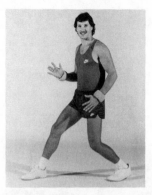
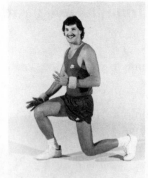

Figure 5-149   Figure 5-150

Cues: Step forward and twist-down; two, three, four; twist-up, two, three, four; walk-through-forward (or backward) and twist, two, three, four; twist-up, two, three, four.

Up, Out, Up, Down Pattern

1

Standing in a medium stride facing diagonally right, thrust chest forward, head high, and bring elbows **up** to shoulder height and out wide to the sides, with hands in fists. Raise right foot to a right toe-touch position by bending right knee. **1 count.**

2

Swing extended arms and fists down to shoulder height and **out** wide to the sides, as head tilts back to a chin-high position. Raise to a two toe-touch position by bending both knees. **1 count.**

3

Repeat step *1*. **1 count.**

4

Taking weight on your left foot, bend ankles, knees, and hips and touch right foot next to left. Bring arms **down** and flexed with fists in to abdomen. Head follows movement down, with a chin toward chest position. **1 count.**

5-8

Reverse pattern by keeping weight on left foot and pivoting forward ending facing diagonally left. Place right foot *back* in a medium-stride position. Repeat gestures of chest thrust, arms **up**-position with left toe-touch (diagonally forward and left), **out, up, down,** finishing with weight on right foot and left toe-touching next to right foot. **4 counts.**

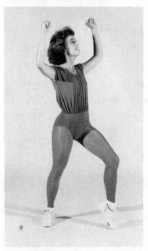
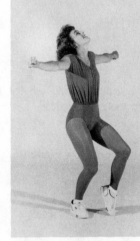

Figure 5-151   Figure 5-152

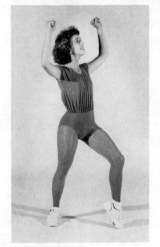
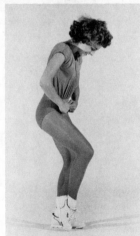

Figure 5-153   Figure 5-154

Cues: Stride and up, out, up, down; pivot-back-stride and up, out, up, down.

Varsity Heel and Toe Strut

1

Facing the right with weight evenly balanced, "**strut**" (step in place) with your left foot. **1 count.**

2

Extending your left arm low and forward while bending and **pulling** your right arm, flex both wrists tightly with palms held in a blade-gesture, facing away; touch right **heel** forward. **1 count.**

3

Strut-step, taking weight backward on the right foot. **1 count.**

4

Bend your left knee and raise the foot to a high toe-**touch** gesture. Alternate arm gestures, with right arm extended and pushing down and left arm held in the bent position. **1 count.**

Cues: Strut, heel and pull; strut, touch and push.

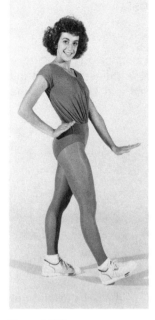 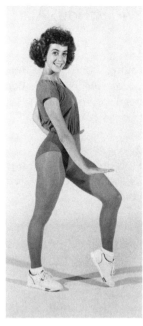

Figure 5-155   **Figure 5-156**

Walk

1

Pace walk forward, starting with the right foot, arms at waist level with elbows bent. **1 count** (each pace walk).

Cues: Pace-walk forward and (count).

For variety, pace **walk:**

—**backward; Cues: Pace-walk-back, and (count).**
—**diagonally** forward or backward; **Cues: Pace-walk-diagonally right, and (count).**
—directly **sideward; Cues: Pace-walk-side, and (count).**
—use **hand weights; Cues: Pace-walk-lift, and (count).**
—a wide variety of **arm gestures** can make this option as exciting as any presented in this text. **Cues: (Arm movements).**

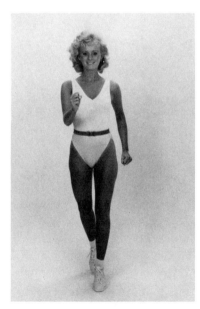

Figure 5-157

Widestride, Arm Crossover

1

Facing front, place the feet comfortably apart in a **widestride** position. **Bending** at the waist, point the head down with arms **crossed** and extended to the floor. **4 counts.**

2

Hold the widestride position and bring the head **up** as the crossed arms remain in front of the body. **4 counts.**

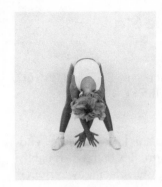

Figure 5-158

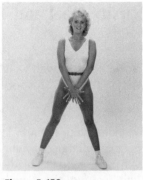

Figure 5-159

3

Hold the widestride position and **raise** crossed arms above head. Look up and away. **4 counts.**

4

Hold the widestride position as the arms extend **out and down** to the sides. (Keep the arms and body very firm throughout the action.) **4 counts.**

Cues: Stride-bend and cross, up, raise, out and down.

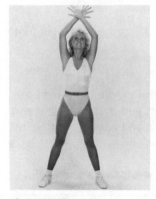

Figure 5-160

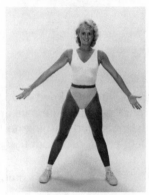

Figure 5-161

X-Pump, Down 'N Up

1

Stand wide**stride** with toes pointing out. Extend arms **down,** out to the sides with palms facing forward and fingers stretched wide in jazz-hand gesture. **1 count.**

2

Bend both knees as you bend elbows with forearms and fingers facing **up. 1 count.**

Cues: Stride and down, bend and up.

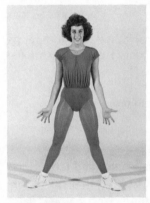

Figure 5-162

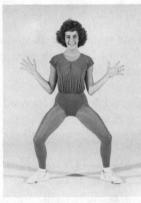

Figure 5-163

Yipee Big 'N Little

1

Jump high, taking off from both feet. At the same time, turn right 90 degrees and **clap** as you land. **1 count.**

2

Jump **in place,** not as high this time, and land. **1 count.**

Repeat **1** and **2** three more times, **turning** 90 degrees each time. End facing front.

Cues: Big, turn-clap, little and clap; turn-clap, little-clap; turn-clap, little-clap; turn front-clap, little-clap.

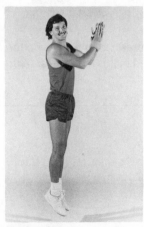

Figure 5-164

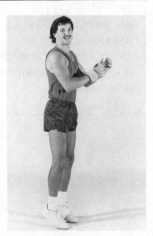

Figure 5-165

Zippity-Do-Dah Pattern

1

Weight begins on your left foot. Swing right leg diagonally forward and **across** left foot and **touch.** Bend left elbow and raise it to shoulder height, with fist at center chest. Right arm and fist are held at right side. **1 count.**

2

Keeping your weight on your left foot, point and **touch** right foot out **wide** to the right side. Right bent elbow raises to shoulder height, fist at chest. Left arm and fist are held at left side. **1 count.**

3

Draw right leg in, take weight on both feet, and **bend** both knees as you reverse arms to the step *1* position. **1 count.**

4

Bring right foot in next to left foot, **straighten** your body to a full stand, and reverse arms to the step *2* position. **1 count.**

Cues: Cross-touch, wide-touch, bend, straighten.

Note: Perfect this coordination pattern in the above described directions before attempting the reverse. Learn the step pattern separately, then the arm gestures separately, and then combine them together.

5-8

Weight is on your right foot. **Cross-touch** left, **wide-touch** left, **bend, straighten.** Begin with right arm bent and left arm down; then alternate this gesture with each step. **4 counts.**

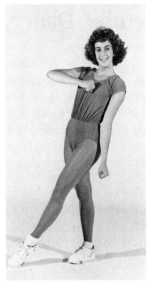 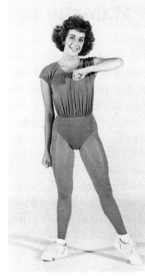

Figure 5-166   **Figure 5-167**

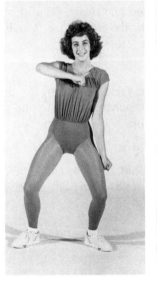 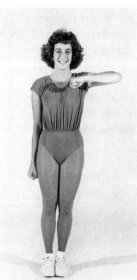

Figure 5-168   **Figure 5-169**

In Conclusion

The coordination skills involved in the Zippity-Do-Dah pattern will be a challenging conclusion to the complete catalogue of gesture and step patterns described in this text. The aforementioned aerobic dance movement possibilities are just the beginnings of a complete listing of creative possibilities you can experience. Continue to increase your aerobic dance A-B-C's by developing **your own** additions to the alphabet. Make a list of any new ideas you create with stick figures and cues.

Catalogue of Aerobic Dance Gesture and Step Pattern Cues

A

"A-B-C-D" Pattern: Fwd, side, back, together (or hold); fwd, side, back, together (or hold).
"A-B-C-D" Sequences: Right fwd 4, side 4, back 4, hold 4; repeat left fwd 4, etc. Right fwd 3 and hold 1, side 3 and hold 1, back 3 and hold 1, hold 4; repeat left fwd 3 and hold 1, etc. Right fwd 2, side 2, back 2, hold 2; repeat left fwd 2, etc. Right fwd, side, back, hold; left fwd, side, back, hold.
Arm Circle: Circle-back.

B

Bounce, Two Feet: Bounce. Or: Lift, bounce.
Bounce, Two Feet Variation: Punch, bounce.
Bounce-Step, Bounce-Touch: Bounce-step, bounce-touch; bounce-step, bounce-touch.
Bounce Steps, With Side Touch: Bounce, touch, bounce, touch.

C

Cha-Cha: Cross, back, step-step, step; cross, back, step-step, step.
Cha-Cha, With Kick Pattern: Cross, back, step, kick, step, step, step-step, step.
Charleston Flapper Walk: Step and swing, lift and swing down; lift and swing, lift and swing down.
Cross-Step Forward, Touch to the Side: Cross, touch; cross, touch.
Cross-Step, Hop: Cross, hop; cross, hop.

D

"Doubles": Knees and Kicks: Knee-lift, down, up, down; kick, down, up, down.
Double Hops: Hop, hop and punch; hop, hop and punch.
Double Hop, Hitch Kick: Hop, hop-kick; hop, hop-kick.

E

Elbow Wipers: Lunge and hold, 2, 3, 4, point, hold, wide, hold, point, hold, wide, hold; walk-through and lunge, (hold) 2, 3, 4, point, hold, wide, hold, point, hold, wide, hold.

F

Fall Back 'N Jump Forward Pattern: Step, step-step, back, forward.

G

Gallop: Step, slide and lift.
Grapevine: Side, back, side, touch; side, back, side, touch.
Grapevine, Varieties:
. . . 'n Kick: Side, back, side, kick.
. . . 'n Hop: Side, back, side, hop-clap (or hop-click, or hop-punch).
. . . 'n Jump-Clap: Side, back, side, jump-clap.

H

Heel-Out, Toe-In Hop Pattern: Out, in, out, jump; out, in, out, jump.
Hip Thrust: Stride, thrust; stride, thrust.
Hop, Kick: Hop, kick; hop, kick.
Hopscotch: Stride, hop, stride, hop.
Hopscotch, Variety: Stride, hop-touch; stride, hop-touch.
Hustle: Jog, jog, jog, lift-clap; jog-back, jog, jog, lift-clap.
. . . Cross-Elbow Touch: Jog, jog, jog, elbow-touch; jog, jog, jog, elbow-touch.
. . . High Impact: Hop, hop, hop, lift; hop, hop, hop, lift.
. . . Low Impact: Pace-walk, walk, walk, lift; pace-walk-back, walk, walk, lift.

I

Itchy-Strut: Step, lift; step, lift.

J
Jazz Touch—Out 'N In Pattern: Out, in, out, shift-your-weight; out, in, out, weight-right.
Jazz Touch—Forward 'N Backward Pattern: Forward, back, forward, shift-your-weight; forward, back, forward, weight-right.
Jazz Walk: Touch-side-wide, swing-click; step, swing-click and cross-touch.
Jazz Side-Walk: Step-side-wide, together.
Jog: Jog—heel first.
. . . Circling: Jog, 2, 3, 4, 5, 6, 7, 8. Jog—left, 2, 3, 4, 5, 6, 7, 8.
Jumps:
. . . One-Foot Jump: Jump-right; jump-left.
. . . Two-Foot Jump: Jump and clap!
. . . Circling: 3 o'clock, 6 o'clock, 9 o'clock, noon; reverse-and-9 o'clock, 6 o'clock, 3 o'clock, 12 o'clock.
. . . Forward 'N Backward: Jump-forward, jump-back.
. . . 'N Land, Widestride: Jump and land-wide, hold.
. . . Side Jump, Clap: Jump-side, clap; side, clap.
. . . Ski Jump: Jump-side, hold; jump-side, hold.
Jumping Jacks:
. . . Regular: Stride-clap, together-slap.
Crazy: Stride, cross; stride, cross.
Double Pattern: X, high I, X, low I.

K
Knee-Lift Elbow-Touch, Varieties:
. . . Same Side: Step-lift, elbow-touch-same; repeat left.
. . . Open to Side: Step-lift, elbow-touch-open; repeat left.
. . . Crossed: Step-lift, cross-elbow-touch; repeat left.
High Intensity: Hop-lift, elbow-touch-(same/open/crossed).

L
Lunges:
. . . Forward: Forward lunge, 2, 3, 4, 5, 6, 7, 8; walk-through-and-lunge, 2, 3, 4, 5, 6, 7, 8.
. . . Scissor: Jump-forward, scissor-jump.
. . . Side: Lunge-side and count (the holding counts).
. . . Side, with Arm Circling: Lunge-3 o'clock, hold; 6 o'clock, hold; 9 o'clock, hold; noon, hold; reverse counterclockwise.
Side-Bounce 'N Sway: Lunge-side and bounce; sway-lunge and bounce.

M
March: Left, right; forward, to-the-rear, side.
Monkey-Jump Pattern: Jump! Forward, right, back, left, forward; forward, left, back, right, forward, jump!

N
Nasty! Strut: Lunge and bend, bounce and flex; lunge and bend, bounce and flex.

O
Opposite Punch 'N Point: Step far and punch, swing-touch and punch.

P
Polka: Hop-step, step-step; hop-step, step-step.
. . . Circling: To-the-right, back, side, forward.
. . . Low-Impact: Step, step, step, hold; step, step, step, hold.
· · · Side-to-Side: To-the-left; to-the-right.
Prance: Touch-push, shift-touch and pull.

Q
Quads 'N Hams Coordination Pattern: Step, lift-front, step, lift-back.

R
Reach: Step, reach; step, reach.
Rock:
...**Big, Forward 'N Backward:** Rock-forward and back.
...**Side-to-Side:** Rock-side; side.
Side-to-Side Variety: Rock-side and punch; side and punch.

S
Shake Up, Shake Down: Shake, two, three, four; shake-down, six, seven, eight.
Skip: Step, hop; step, hop.
Slides: Step, together-step.
Slide, Bend, Jump, Clap Pattern: Slide, bend, jump, clap; slide, bend, jump, clap.
Snob Strut: Side-step and touch, snob and bounce; twist and touch, snob and bounce.
Step, Hop: Step, hop.
...**Circling:** Step, hop to the side; step, hop to the back; step, hop to the side; step, hop front.
Step, Hop, Step, Kick Pattern: Step, hop, step, kick.
Step, Kick: Step, kick; step, kick.
...**Circling:** Step, kick; two; three; four; five; six; seven; eight.
...**'N Punch-Down:** Step, kick-side and punch down, step, kick-front and punch down.
...**Sidekick:** Step, side-kick and click; step, side-kick and click.
Step, Lift, Touch, Lift Pattern: Step, lift, touch, lift; step, lift, touch, lift.
Stride 'N Twist Pattern: Stride, cross, turn, hold, lift, touch, kick, touch.

T
The Twist: Step forward and twist-down, 2, 3, 4; twist-up, 2, 3, 4; walk-through-forward (or back) and twist, 2, 3, 4; twist-up, 2, 3, 4.

U
Up, Out, Up, Down Pattern: Stride and up, out, up, down; pivot-back-stride and up, out, up, down.

V
Varsity Heel 'N Toe Strut: Strut, heel and pull; strut, touch and push.

W
Walk: Pace-walk-forward and (count each pace walk).
Walk Varieties, with Creative Arm Gestures:
...**Backward:** Pace-walk back and (count).
...**Diagonally:** Pace-walk diagonally-right, and (count).
...**Sideward:** Pace-walk-side, and (count).
...**with Hand Weights:** Pace-walk-lift, and (count).
Widestrides:
...**Arm Crossover:** Stride-bend and cross, up, raise, out and down.

X
X-Pump, Down 'N Up: Stride and down (arms), bend and up (arms).

Y
Yippee Big 'N Little: Big, turn-clap, little and clap; turn-clap, little-clap; turn-clap, little-clap; turn-front-clap, little-clap.

Z
Zippity-Do-Dah Pattern: Cross-touch, wide-touch, bend, straighten; cross-touch, wide-touch, bend, straighten.

6

THE COOL-DOWN:
Catalogue of Exercises and
A Routine

Purpose of the Cool-Down

The purpose of a planned cool-down portion of your hour is to give your body time to readjust back to the pre-activity state in which you began. This will ease the gradual process of returning the large quantity of blood that is now in your working muscles (primarily your arms and legs) back toward your head and trunk (brain and other vital organs). An abrupt stopping of a highly strenuous activity session may cause the blood (primarily in your legs) to "pool" or stay in the extremities. This will occur because the veins of the legs are not being forcefully squeezed now by strenuously working leg muscles.

The result of this "pooling" can cause cramping, nausea, dizziness, and/or fainting, since the needed quantity of oxygen and blood is not being delivered to the brain and other vital organs. So do not forget this very important last phase.

What Determines the Time?

Your ability to recover from exertion will usually determine how long of a cool-down you will need to include. A **minimum of five minutes** is essential, however, for two reasons:

- To curtail profuse sweating.

- To lower the heart rate to below 120 beats per minute.

These are two visible signs to monitor and achieve before concluding your exercise hour.

Cool-Down Is Gradual

You'll begin your cooling down process with a complete **slowing down of all large muscle activity.** Tapering off your activity level can be performed in various ways: slow dancing, slow walking, etc. This kind of activity begins the transition between the vigorous activity just completed and the **cool-down stretching that you perform last.**

Stretching as a Conclusion to Your Program

Equally important to the warm-up stretching preceding an aerobic dance workout are the cool-down stretching exercises that immediately follow the program.

Cool-down stretching has a twofold purpose:

- To further provide needed time for your body to

readjust from strenuous exertion.
- To further increase your flexibility at a prime time when your muscles and connective tissues are warm and supple.

Here are a few guidelines to follow to make your stretching portion of the cool-down an enjoyable experience:

1
You first assume a sitting position and begin independent or choreographed slow stretches to background music.

2
The music chosen should be slow-tempoed, low-key type music that suggests or promotes relaxation.

3
Remember, however, that during the cool-down phase you are **not completely relaxing** your muscles yet—you are **purposefully tightly stretching** and releasing (relaxing) the stretch.

4
Cool-down stretch every muscle group and joint you just used during the hour.

5
Stretching is completed in a lying down position. At the conclusion of stretching in the lying position, your legs are then elevated and held stretched skyward to ease (and hasten) the return of venous blood from your legs back to your heart.

Note: A mental relaxation technique would then follow to conclude your entire workout hour and provide a refreshing conclusion to your total stress-release program. This information is presented in Chapter 7.

Cool-Down Stretching

Here is a summary of key points:
- Taper off large muscle activity gradually by first dancing or walking slowly.
- Controlled stretching follows and is begun in a sitting position.
- Low-key, slow music is an excellent accompaniment to cool-down stretching.
- Remember to breathe constantly. Exhale as you stretch and hold; inhale as you recover.
- Complete your stretching sequence in a lying down position, ending your physical exercise program with legs elevated skyward.

A Cool-Down Stretching Routine

The following stretching routine incorporates all of the suggested guidelines to encourage not only the return of blood to your head and central trunk and eliminate the excess from your arms and legs, but also to promote and increase your flexibility. Remember—the cool-down provides the "safety valve" after aerobics or strength training (i.e., strenuous activity) and is an absolute **must!**

Directions

Again, continue in the **last** position when a new exercise begins, unless noted to change; perform all the exercises as you **see** them shown.

1
You begin the cool-down with **slow dancing** and **walking** movements. Perform this first exercise as you either slow dance an in-place continual **side-touch**, or **standing wide-stride**; or as you slowly walk around the perimeter of the room.

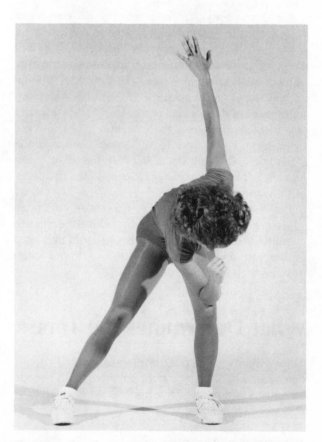

Figure 6-0. Slow dancing and walking to begin cool-down.

Snaps—Up/Down/Across

1

Extend arms forward and parallel, shoulder high, fists facing. **2 counts.**

2

Bend forearms toward you, keeping elbows still forward and shoulder high; **click** fingers above you. **2 counts.**

3

Return arms forward and click fingers. **2 counts.**

4

For variety, try arms working in opposition, one forward and clicking, and one bent and clicking. Alternate. **4 counts.**

5

Lower elbows to sides, keeping forearms high and parallel. **Snap. 2 counts.**

6

Extend forearms down, to straight-arm and parallel position and **snap. 2 counts.**

7

Extend arms **out** to the side, shoulder high. **Snap** here. **2 counts.**

8

Swing arms down, **cross-chest** and **snap. 2 counts.**

9

Swing back **out** to shoulder high position. **Snap. 2 counts.**

10

Swing arms **down** and **behind** buttocks and **snap. 2 counts.**

11

Swing arms back **out** to shoulder high position. **Snap. 2 counts.**

Cues: **Extend, bend and click; bend and extend, alternate; lower elbows, snap, extend, snap; out, snap, cross-chest, snap, out, snap, down-behind, snap, out, snap.**

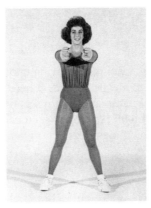

Figure 6-1.

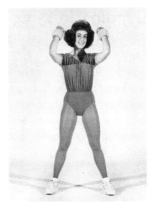

Figure 6-2.

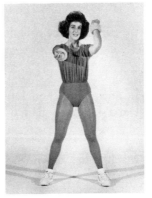

Figure 6-3.

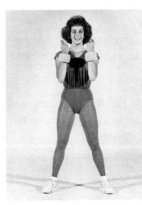

Figure 6-4.

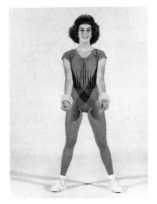

Figure 6-5.

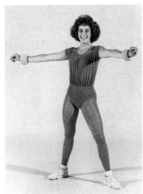

Figure 6-6.

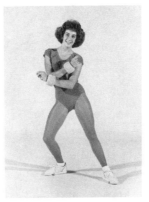

Figure 6-7.

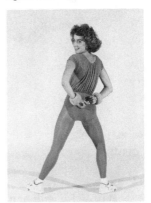

Figure 6-8.

Standing To Lying Transition

1

Conclude the walking or slow dancing by moving into one large circle facing in; or, to any floor space where you have enough room to lie and stretch arms and legs in any direction. **Sit tall** with legs together, toes skyward. Hold arms parallel above legs, shoulder high. **8 counts.**

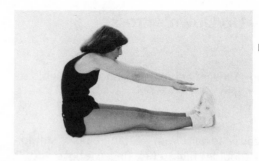

Figure 6-9.

2

Press forward, **reaching** palms over toes in a **chin-lead** position and **hold. 4 counts.**

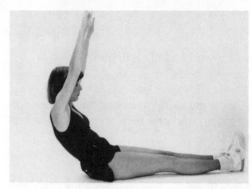

Figure 6-10.

3

Extending arms skyward, slowly **curl down** by rounding your back, with chin to chest, and hold. **8 counts.**

4

Lie tightly **stretched**, with your fingers stretched and pointed and your toes tightly flexed skyward and hold. **4 counts.**

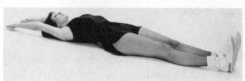

Figure 6-11.

Cues: Sit tall, press and reach, curl down, lie stretched.

Knee-Lift (Hamstring Stretch)

1

Bring one **knee to chest** with toe pointed. Keep other leg straight in position, with toe flexed and hold. **4 counts.**

4

Bring **two knees up** to chest. Encircle upper shins with hands and arms, keeping toes pointed. Pull knees down to chest and **hold. 8 counts.**

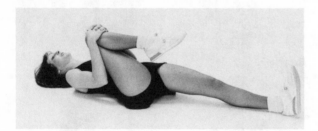

Figure 6-12.

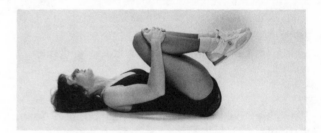

Figure 6-13.

2

Relax leg back to the floor 4 counts and **stretch. 4 counts.**

3

Repeat exercise with **opposite knee to chest** followed by **relaxing** leg back to the floor and **stretch. 12 counts.**

Cues: Knee to chest, relax and stretch; other knee to chest, relax and stretch; two knees up, hold.

One-Leg Cross-Over (Waist)

1

Uncurl extended leg back down to floor, and **stretch arms** resting on floor **shoulder high** or higher; keep toes flexed and hold. **8 counts.**

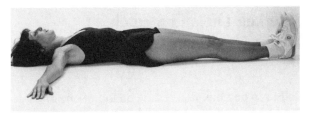

Figure 6-14.

2

Raise **one leg skyward** with ankle flexed, keeping other leg on floor and tightly flexed at ankle and hold. **4 counts.**

3

Keeping arms and chest **on** floor, **lower** raised leg **across body** to floor near your outstretched opposite palm and hold. **8 counts.**

4

Raise same leg skyward and **lower** to floor and hold. **8 counts.**

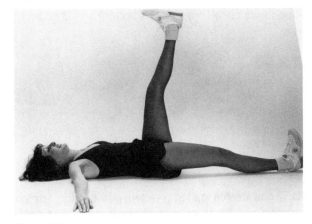

Figure 6-15.

5

Repeat entire sequence with **opposite** leg. **20 counts.**

Cues: Stretch arms shoulder high; one leg skyward, lower across body; raise; lower. Repeat opposite leg.

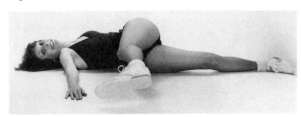

Figure 6-16.

Butt-Tucks (Buttocks)

1

Lie on back with knees skyward. Place feet one foot from buttocks and six inches apart. Arms are at your sides on the floor. Breathe easy. **4 counts.**

2

Slowly exhale and with stomach tightly contracted, **lift** buttocks to the ''up'' position and hold tightly contracted for 8 seconds. Be sure upper back and shoulders are taking the body weight (and **not** your cervical spine) and also that your feet are flat on the floor. Breathe easy and continuously. **8 counts.**

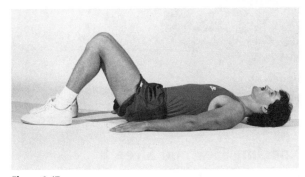

Figure 6-17.

3

Slowly inhale and **lower** buttocks to floor. **8 counts.**

Repeat 4 times. **64 counts.**

Cues: Lift, lower.

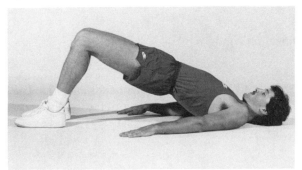

Figure 6-18.

Side Leg Lift and Stretch
(Inner Thigh and Calf)

1

Roll onto one hip, legs resting on top of one another. Support body in this position by your top arm, which is in front of your waist area, with palm on floor. Support your head with palm of bottom arm. **8 counts.**

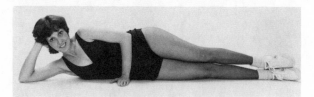

Figure 6-19.

2

Raise and stretch top leg skyward, pointing toe; stretch top arm and hand, pointing toward ankle, and hold. **4 counts. Lower** leg. **4 counts.**

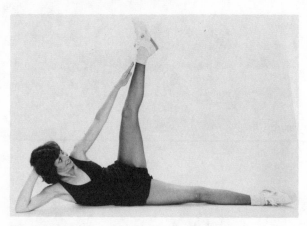

Figure 6-20.

3

Repeat slow raising and lowering three more times. **24 counts.**

4

Roll onto your **back side** (supine), and then onto **opposite hip. Repeat** the entire sequence four times. **40 counts.**

Cues: Raise and stretch; lower.

5 Advanced

Rest body weight on your bottom bent elbow and forearm. Bend knee that is on the floor (leg extending backward). **Raise** top leg, grasp toe, and tightly flex and **pull** leg toward you. **8 counts.**

Figure 6-21.

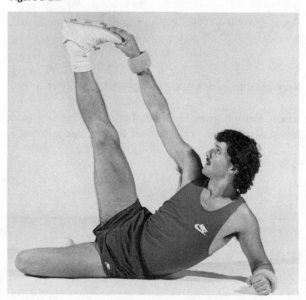

Cues: Raise and pull.

Kneeling Flex and Stretch
(Spine, Buttocks, Legs)

1

Kneel on hands and knees. **4 counts.**

2

Bring head down as right knee **bends** inward toward the chest. As your head and knee come together, **hold. 4 counts.**

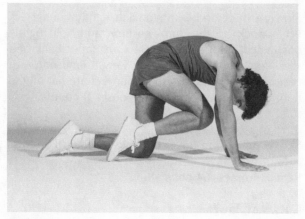

Figure 6-22.

3

Lift and extend head forward and leg backward, directly in a straight line with your spine. **4 counts.**

4

Repeat 4 times. **32 counts.**

5

Return to kneeling on both knees and alternate with flexing and stretching left leg 4 times. **32 counts.**

Cues: Flex and stretch.

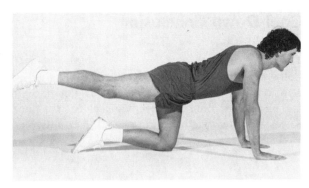

Figure 6-23.

Hydrant-Lift (Inner Thigh, Buttocks)

1

Weight is still evenly balanced on all fours, head forward. **Lift** your right knee directly out to the right side. Knee is bent and lifted to hip height, thigh parallel to the floor, arms **firm. 4 counts.**

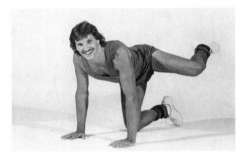

Figure 6-24.

2

Lower right knee directly down, but not touching the floor. **4 counts.**

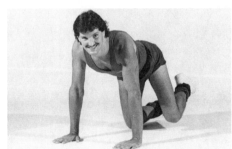

Figure 6-25.

3

Repeat 4 times. **32 counts.**

4

Alternate and perform with the left knee to the left side. Repeat 4 times. **32 counts.**

5

Progressively over time, add a one, two, or three pound weight to the ankle of the lifting leg. Maintain firm arms and a flat stable spine, with abdominals tightly tucked. Don't give in to a "swayback" position!

Low-Back Stretch (Spine, Knees)

1

Continue in the same position, kneeling on your hands and knees with weight evenly distributed, back straight, abdominals pulled in, and head in line with spine. **4 counts.**

2

Sit back on your heels and lower your chest against your thighs. Keep your hands in place on the floor in front of you and drop your head. Hold position **12 counts.**

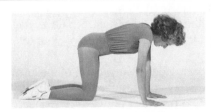

Figure 6-26.

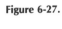

Figure 6-27.

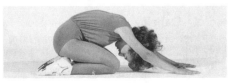

Cues: Kneel, sit back.

Cool-Down Conclusion

1
Roll onto your back side again, and place outstretched arms on floor, shoulder high with palms down. Slide feet in toward buttocks, keeping feet flat on floor. Knees are now together and skyward. **8 counts.**

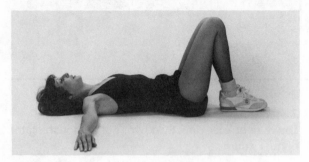

Figure 6-28.

2
Pull both knees to chest. **4 counts.**

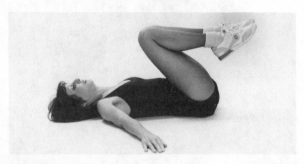

Figure 6-29.

3
Extend legs skyward, keeping knees slightly flexed. Hold position approximately one minute—**120 counts.** Remember to continuously breathe now. This will hasten the blood supply in the legs, back to the central trunk area.

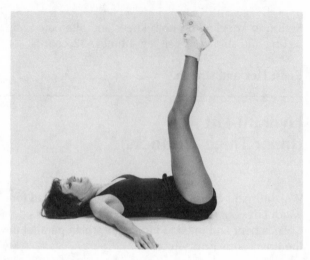

Figure 6-30.

4
Lower legs to the floor and proceed with relaxation techniques; or, begin the strength development phase of your program.

Cool-Down Summary

The statistics reflect that if a problem is going to most likely occur in an aerobic dance program, it will most frequently occur **during the cool-down phase.** This is the time frame when all of the bodily systems are readjusting to the pre-activity state. So, never neglect this all-important **five to ten minutes** of your total fitness program.

The following is an index review of all of the cool-down exercises which were presented in this chapter, in **sequential-routine order:**

- Slow Dancing in Place with Side Touch, Wide-Stride, or Walking Perimeter of Room.
- Snaps—Up/Down/Cross
- Standing to Lying Transition
- Knee-Lift
- One-Leg Cross-Over
- Butt-Tucks
- Side-Leg—Lift and Stretch
- Kneeling Flex and Stretch
- Hydrant-Lift
- Low-Back Stretch
- Cool-Down Conclusion

Strength Development

If you are interested in incorporating a strength program during your aerobic dance hour, **now** is the time in your workout program to do so.

Strength activities are performed to more quickly "define," "tone," "shape," make more dense, **i.e., thicken** your muscle fibers. It will also allow you to **endure longer** periods of work—both during your exercise workout program, and later, in your daily work tasks.

A general strengthening of all of the muscles of the body occurs during vigorous aerobic dance. However, a strength program that is included within an aerobic dance hour that focuses on the strength development of **isolated muscle groups** (i.e., the chest, abdomen, lower legs, upper arms) is performed at the **end** of the aerobic dance workout.

The reasoning for this is simple. With an increase in the resistance (weights) that must be applied to any movement for significant change (i.e., "training") to occur, there is also an increase in the workload that is placed on the heart, lungs, and vascular system. An individual is more readily, therefore, placed in a breathless, "oxygen-debt" state.

During the aerobic dancing phase, your goal is **not** to be in a breathless state. You want to be continually working in a breathe-easy state, steadily pacing your intensity.

Also, with the addition of free weights, being able to **safely control the range of motion that all of the joints will experience** (i.e., the knees, spine, etc.) is vitally important, so that injuries do not occur. Aerobic dance movement is dynamic, covering space, and it is not easy to continuously control a wide variety of movement with heavy weights in hand.

So, save the specific, isolated muscle-group strength exercises until the final phase of your workout hour. And, follow the principles and guidelines established for strength training. Here are a few basics to remember:

- Muscle strengthening exercises should be **preceded and followed by stretching** exercises that are specific for the muscles that are made to work against resistance. And, any muscle group strengthened by exercise should also be regularly stretched to prevent abnormal contraction of resting length.[1]
- You can use your body's weight against gravity as a "resistance" ("weights used") as in push-ups or curl-ups. **Note:** Your head can be an extremely heavy weight when used during exercise. Anytime it is brought forward and flexed (as in a forehead reaching, chin-tucked position), it is considered an **advanced only** position and only for individuals who are quite flexible and strong in the cervical spine (neck) area. To progressively increase the resistance involved in lifting your body's weight against gravity, a strategically placed free-weight is used (ie., on the sternum for a curl-up, between the shoulder blades for a push-up, etc.).

- All strengthening exercises should be performed in a slow and controlled manner. Ballistic (rapid or jerky) movements increase the risk of injury.[1]
- Repeat the move ("repetitions") with excellent, full range-of-motion form, as many times as possible. (Your "set.") **When the form of your "set" declines** and you become jerky, are not rhythmical in the move, and are not using the full range of motion possible around your joints, you've completed your lower limit possible of the set! Make a record of this number. This lower limit becomes your baseline to which you attempt to add more repetitions as early as possible. Repetitions should, however, be limited to short sets (ten or fewer) that are repeated later.[1]

  And, it will later be **less** beneficial if just more repetitions are performed without adding additional external weight (i.e., using a heavier free weight). Adding weights, in one-pound increments at a time, will provide the added resistance you need over the long-range course of your program.

- From the wide variety of exercise movements pictured and described in this text—whether listed as warm-up stretching, aerobic dance gesture and step patterns, or cool-down stretching movements—**all** of these can be possibilities for your free-weight strength program. It is simply a matter of adding a hand or leg weight, slowly controlling the movement, and then repeating the movement for approximately four to eight repetitions with each side of the body, arm, or leg. The choice of accompanying music must be of a slow tempo, however.

  Thus, variety is the "spice" of any program. You will never lack for ideas if you incorporate other movements that you already know. **Steady control** in performing these moves is the key! This means for the aerobic gesture and step patterns you will want to avoid the high impact movements of jumping, hopping, jogging, etc. You will perform instead at low impact (i.e., floor contact) movement like touches, bounces, and walk steps.

- Strength training using weights and repetitions for isolated muscle groups is performed on an **every other day** basis. Your muscles need a day to recover, so don't incorporate a program to strength train with weights daily.

  An alternative to this program is to perform strength training exercises with hand/wrist weights for the **upper half of your body one day**, and use leg/ankle weights and perform exercises for the **lower half of your body the next day.** You are thus alternating the days that the muscles are strength training.

- The most efficient way to improve strength is to allow brief **rest periods between bouts** of vigorous exercise.[1]
- Finally, just remember to begin your program slowly, methodically, and in absolute control of the amount of weights you are using. Strength-fitness training to more fully develop muscle strength and endurance is a long-term project[2] calling for a dedicated personal commitment of many hours, just as the programs of stretching for flexibility improvement, and aerobics for aerobic capacity improvement are. **All fitness programs are for life!**

Strength Training Exercises

The following are strength training exercises which include work on each major muscle group of the body. They utilize a variety of means:

- Your own weight against gravity.
- Heavy Hands or dumbbells held in the hands.
- Wrist or ankle weights worn over those joints.

Perform the following exercises and then record your results as "strength training after aerobic dance." Include the following in your recordkeeping: the date, weight resistance used if any, number of repetitions you performed in excellent form, and the number of sets you performed.

Bent Knee Curl-Ups (Abdomen)

1

Since these muscles are key muscles responsible for assisting in holding the body upright, strong abdominals are a **must** to avoid overstressing the opposing muscle groups of the back, along the spinal column.

2

Lying on the floor in a supine position, lay your hands across your chest. Bend your knees and place your feet **flat** on the floor, about one foot from your buttocks. (The angle of your lower legs to your thighs will be approximately 90 degrees.) Always do curl-ups in this position, to protect the lower back.

3

A partner can kneel at your feet and secure your feet in the flat position by placing weight and hands on your shoe-toes or ankle area.

4

Rounding your spine with chin to chest, curl up, keeping feet flat on the floor. Your forehead will be above your knees. **4 counts.**

5

A full curl-up is counted when you have rounded your back, smoothly raised your trunk until your lower back is perpendicular to the floor, and then have curled and returned back down to the lying position.[3] **8 counts.**

6

Smooth curling up and down in a **slow, rhythmical form** is the goal you desire. Performing this exercise

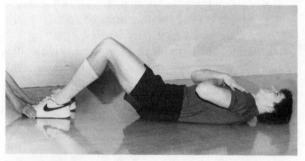

Figure 6-31. Step 1—lying.

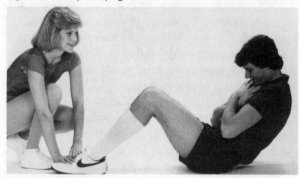

Figure 6-32. Step 2—curling.

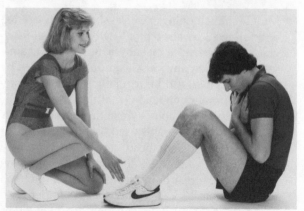

Figure 6-33. Step 3—up.

with speed will encourage slamming the back to the floor, or not using a full range of motion.

Cues: Exhale and curl up, inhale and curl down.

7
Persons who lack stomach strength will tend to move feet out and away from buttocks. **Try to avoid this**, keeping feet in close to buttocks, with knees bent at a 90-degree angle (lower legs to thighs).

8
Use your hands and arms to help you curl up if you cannot do the following exercise without using them. Lie with arms at your sides, knees skyward. Put your hands under your thighs to help pull yourself up. Place chin on chest and then meet chin to knees. **4 counts.**

9
Uncurl by rounding the back slowly and lying down. **4 counts.** Be sure to keep feet flat on the floor. Have your partner assist you by holding your feet down if necessary. Repeat until movement becomes jerky and then stop. Increase gradually up to twenty reps. Then try the regular Bent-Knee Curl-Ups.

10   Advanced
Progressively over time place a one- to five-pound weight on sternum (breastbone) area. The weight stays **in contact** with the body on the curl-up.

Caution: If the muscles start to quiver and you feel yourself lifting and jerking to get up instead of easily curling the back, STOP. This indicates that the abdominal muscles are tired and will transfer the work to the lower back muscles, possibly causing lower back pain.

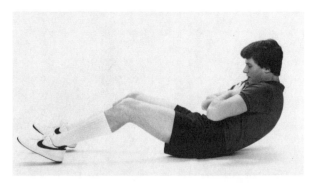

Figure 6-34. Do not move feet out.

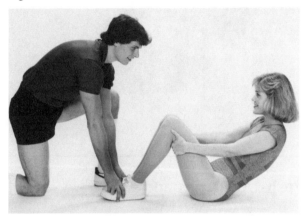

Figure 6-35.

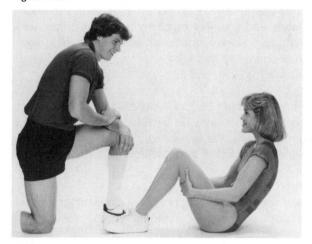

Figure 6-36.

Leg-High Curl-Ups (Abdomen)

1
Stretch your legs skyward, knees slightly bent. Place hands **across** your chest. **4 counts.**

2
Exhale, and **lift** your head, neck, and upper back using your abdominal muscles to pull you up, chin leading. **4 counts.**

3
Inhale and release abdominal muscles and **curl back** to the floor, keeping legs stabilized. **4 counts.**

4
Exhale and lift to **curl up** even **farther**, by stretching your straight arms past your extended legs, knees-bent position. **4 counts.**

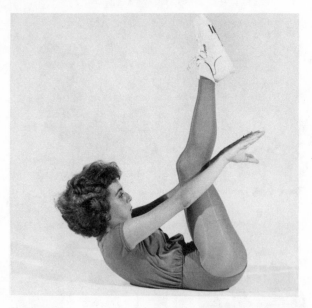

Figure 6-37.

5
Repeat *3*, **curl back. 4 counts.**

Cues: Cross and stretch; lift, curl back, curl up farther, curl back.

Push-Ups (Arms and Chest)

1
Push-ups are often done as fast as possible. Try them **slowly** and see how much more effective they are! Perform **4 slow counts down and exhale,** then **four slow counts up and inhale.**

2
Your feet should be 2 to 4 inches apart. For beginner push-ups, knees are on the floor, with legs extended directly back. For advanced, weight is on the toes, with knees relaxed and not locked.

3
Your fingers should be spread and pressing the ground so undue strain is not felt in the wrists.

4
Your elbows should be neither locked when your arms are fully extended to begin with, nor overbent when at the lowest part of the push-up.

5
Align your head straight out from your shoulders. Don't raise it up or drop it below a straight line.

6
Your buttocks should be a little up, out of line with the rest of your body, and in order to protect your low back.[4] Stomach muscles must be held in tight and not be relaxed and pushing out.

For Beginners

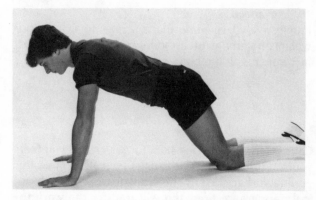

Figure 6-38.

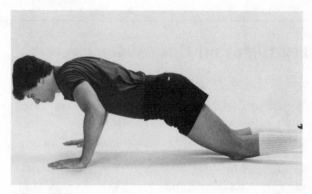

Figure 6-39.

7

The number of push-ups you perform depends upon the muscle strength and endurance in your chest and arms. Initially record how many you can perform **continuously, and maintaining the good form described, without stopping.** When your form begins to deteriorate or when you get tired, rest, and recover your breath. Attempt one or two more sets of these repetitions. Your (endurance) goal is to increase the number of repetitions. The speed at which you perform them should remain slow and constant, taking 8 counts per push-up.

8

For developing more strength, advanced persons can place a weight disk between the shoulder blades while performing the repetitions.

Cues: Exhale and down; inhale and up.

For Advanced

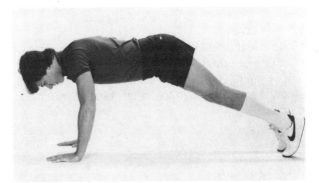

Figure 6-40.

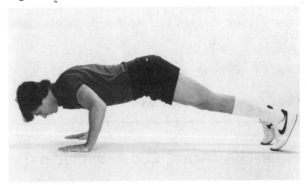

Figure 6-41.

Dumbbell Side Bends
(Obliques, Waist)

A lighter weight (i.e., two to four pounds) with higher repetitions is used for this exercise, since you want to primarily develop tone and muscle endurance in this waist area muscle.

1

Hold a wrist weight or have a dumbbell in each hand at sides, palms facing each other inward.

2

Bend slowly down to one side as far as possible, trying to touch the outside of the knee while lowering weight. Dumbbell in other hand can be (a) raised to waist high level; (b) left hanging at your side; or (c) omitted, using no weight in opposite hand. Pause. **4 counts.**

3

Return to starting position. **4 counts.**

4

Alternate and bend to the other side as far as possible, pause, and return to starting position. **8 counts.** This completes one rep.

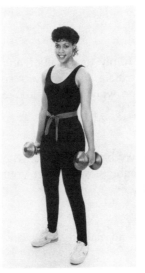

Figure 6-42.

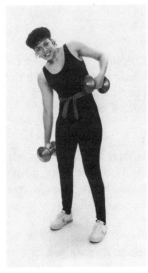

Figure 6-43.

5

Perform two sets of ten reps and work up to two sets of fifteen reps, unless more reps are desired.

Cues: Side bend, return; alternate side-bend, return.

Triceps Extension (Triceps)

1
Grasp one dumbbell with both hands (side by side or atop one another). Raise dumbbell over your head and, keeping upper arm stationary while bending elbow, **lower** dumbbell to directly behind your neck. **4 counts.**

2
Raise weight so that arms are extended skyward. Pause. **4 counts.**

3
Slowly **lower** to behind-the-neck position. **4 counts.**

4
Repeat performing three sets of eight reps.

Cues: Lower; raise and lower.

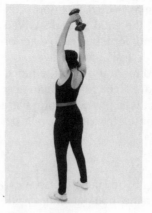
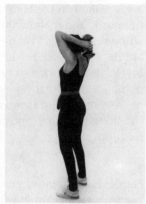

Figure 6-44.   Figure 6-45.

Floor Flys (Arms, Chest, Shoulders)

1
Lie on your back now, knees bent skyward, arms stretched sideward, directly across from shoulders. Place a one- to five-pound weight in each hand, **palms up.**

2
Keeping your back pressed firmly to the floor and keeping your arms straight, **exhale** and slowly **raise** your hands **skyward** until the weights meet above you. **4 counts.**

3
Inhale, and keeping your lower back in contact with the floor and your arms straight, slowly **lower** your hands **to the floor. 4 counts.**

4
Repeat 8 times. Relax, regain normal breathing, and repeat 2 more sets of 8 reps.

Cues: Lie with palms up; exhale and raise skyward, inhale and lower to the floor.

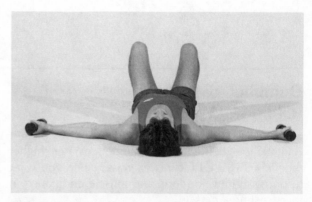

Figure 6-46.

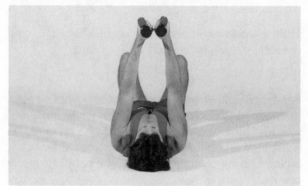

Figure 6-47.

Leg-Flys (Inner Thighs)

1
Remain lying down on your back, with arms on the floor, palms down, shoulder level. **Raise** your **legs** skyward, toes pointed to the **12 o'clock** position.

2
Exhale and open legs to an **11/1 o'clock** position. **4 counts. Inhale and return** to center. **4 counts.**

3
Exhale and open legs as wide as you can, to the **10/2 o'clock position**, if possible. **4 counts. Inhale and return** legs slowly upward, **holding** at each former position. **8 counts.**

4
Some individuals who are extremely flexible will be able to achieve the **9/3 o'clock** position. But for many of us, this extreme is not possible because of the limitations of our flexibility.

Cues: Exhale and open—11/1 o'clock; inhale and return. Exhale and open—10/2 o'clock; inhale and return.

5
Flex feet and repeat.

6
Bring legs past the perpendicular and cross legs at ankles in both pointed and toe-flexion positions.

7 Advanced
Progressively over time, add one-, two-, or three-pound ankle weights. Be sure to keep good position (**lower back always** contacting the floor) and remember to **exhale** as you **open** legs and **inhale** as you **return** them.

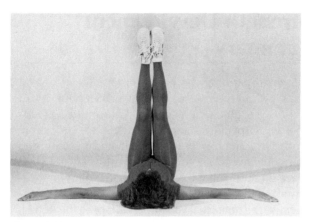
Figure 6-48.

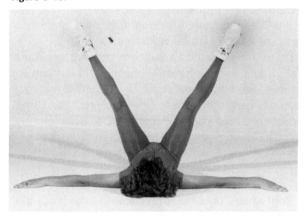
Figure 6-49.

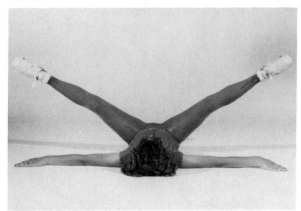
Figure 6-50.

Ankle Flexion (Lower Front Leg)

This exercise is pictured and described in Chapter 11 under "Care and Prevention of Shin Splints."

Note: Follow any and all strength training exercises with another brief cool-down period, adhering to the principles and guidelines presented earlier for a proper cool-down.

Strength Development Summary

Strength training can help you to achieve several goals, within the aerobic dance workout hour. It can assist in beautifully toning all of your muscle groups (that is, **if** specific strength training exercises are included in your program for each isolated muscle group that you want to improve, i.e., chest, legs, stomach, arms, etc.). It can make these muscle groups well-defined and "look better"—more appealing to the eye—because the fibers that you have, have been thickened. And it can provide you with the ability to not only perform difficult (or easy) aerobic dance moves, but also will enable you to perform them over, and over, and over again (muscle endurance).

These are goals that a **strength training program** within your aerobic dance workout can help you to achieve. So, **enjoy** how physically attractive you can become, performing these types of exercises during the last phase of your physical exercise program.

The following is an index review of all of the strength training exercises which were presented in this chapter, in **sequential-routine** order:

- Bent Knee Curl-Ups: Arms Cross Chest; Hands Behind Thighs; Using Weights
- Leg High Curl-Ups: Bent Knees
- Push-Ups: From Knees; From Toes
- Dumbbell Side Bends
- Triceps Extension
- Floor Flys
- Leg Flys: Feet Pointed; Feet Flexed; Feet Crossed; Using Weights
- Ankle Flexion Using Weights

Cool-Down and Strength Development Conclusion

Record any new cool-down stretching and strength exercise activities you may develop. Creating variety in your program with new exercise ideas will counteract boredom!

This concludes a complete physical exercise program. Remember, to be "complete," you need to train in all physical fitness component areas (as depicted in the fitness triangle) every week. This includes a warm-up of stretching (daily), your favorite variety of aerobic conditioning like dancing, jogging, jumping rope, etc. (every other day is good), a strength and muscular endurance routine (every other day), and cool-down movement and stretching after every bout of strenuous exercise. You now hold the key to fitness for a lifetime!

7

RELAXATION and STRESS MANAGEMENT

*"When you can get in touch with an inner
quietness—
A mental pool of renewed energy—
Who then can possibly enter?"*

Developing **total control** of your mind and body is an awesome goal and one for which we all strive, consciously or unconsciously. It seems to take the gift of supreme self-discipline, with which few of us are intuitively blessed, to master total control with ease. Most of us must therefore "work at it" by educating our bodies and minds first. Only through the repetitious practice of all the skill we wish to master will we obtain the self-discipline. This is true for attaining either total physical control or total mental control. **Repetition and practice** are the keys to the total control for which we strive.

Developing total control of our minds to allow us to master relaxation sounds like a uniquely powerful skill. And it can be—**if** you allow yourself the time to learn and practice this skill. For total relaxation **is a skill** that must be mastered. A few individuals may be able to totally relax without any training—but even those few can sharpen their skills with new creative methods and ideas.

You've Earned It—Let's Relax

Have you ever enjoyed an exercise session and left all hot, sweaty, and tired—but happy, just knowing you've done something positive for yourself? Have you, likewise, ever thought how terrific it would be to leave just happy, minus the hot, sweaty, and tired feeling? If so, you've probably never realized that there is another step, or routine procedure, that you need to do to completely reverse the process in which you've just engaged. It allows you to totally eliminate the hot, sweaty, and tired feelings. You instead leave with a feeling of renewed energy. It's called being "energized." All this and no shower yet!

Very simply, here is what happens to your body following sustained, strenuous (not light) exercise, like aerobically dancing, jogging, or jumping rope (i.e., continuously for twenty or more minutes):

1
Beta endorphins, which are natural brain hormones (neuropeptides) with effects similar to those of morphine, and which play a major (but not total) role in the body's control of pain,[1] are released. These hormones then travel from the brain to the spinal fluid and subsequently to all nervous tissue. (Again, this has been found to occur only during sustained physical exertion—not just any light exercise session.)

2
All body nervous tissues receive these natural hormone drugs that have been produced and released, and a glow envelops you. The feeling is described as a "natural high."

3
Your heart rate following the cool-down exercises/routine will lower to approximately the rate taken during the warm-up stretching portion of the hour, and breathing will be easier.

4

Most of the sweating mechanism will begin to subside.

It is now time to incorporate three to fifteen minutes of total relaxation into your fitness program. During this time, the tension previously held in all muscle groups is eliminated as much as possible. You can master this goal with practice in a minimum of approximately two or three minutes.[2] The training period to allow you to master the technique of relaxation will take about five or ten minutes at the conclusion of each aerobic dance session for approximately ten weeks. (When relaxation is practiced before going to bed, or during the middle of the day, fifteen minutes is suggested.) It is easier for beginners to attempt relaxation through practice **after** a sustained exercise session, rather than during or after various daily activities.[3]

You will usually find at the conclusion of this technique that:

1

Your sweating mechanism will have completely stopped.

2

Your breathing rate and body temperature will be back to your normal range.

3

Your heart rate will most likely be lower than when you arrived, and for many will even be approaching (or at) your resting heart rate![4]

All of this with only three minutes of effort following the cool-down!

Voluntary Conscious Relaxation Technique

This technique differs greatly from many other equally effective methods. It totally uses your powers of control through your imagination—your mind seeks out and recognizes tension. It then eliminates it, again through your ability to imagine the relaxation. No physical exertion or planned tensing of muscle groups is performed.

There are four steps to voluntary conscious relaxation:

1

Establishing the relaxation position.

2

Establishing the breathing pattern.

3

"Tuning in" to various parts of the body.

4

Heart rate monitoring followed by simple static stretching to make each person alert again (unless the technique is used prior to going to bed).

Step 1: Establishing the Relaxation Position

1

Lie on your back (Figure 7-1). If you feel uncomfortable because your entire back is not in contact with the floor, raise one knee up with your foot flat on the floor, approximately one foot from your buttocks (Figure 7-2). Persons with either substantial buttocks or shoulder mass will find that this "knee up" position will relieve the arched lower back feeling.

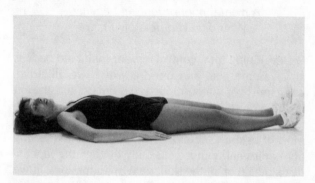

Figure 7-1.

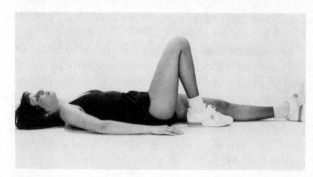

Figure 7-2.

2

Turn your head slightly to one side. When you become totally relaxed, your tongue will relax backward and cover your windpipe if you keep your head straight in line with the rest of you.

3

Place your arms on the floor at your sides, palms down, with elbows a little bent. Flexed joints are more relaxed.

4

Place your legs a bit apart (not crossed or in contact with one another). As the legs relax, your feet will tend to roll outward.

5

If you consciously relax best with your eyes open, keep them open. If you consciously relax best with your eyes closed, close them. If you keep them open, focus **continuously** on **one** object only.

Step 2: Establishing the Breathing Pattern

1

Take a deep breath and hold it in your lungs. Focus in on the chest-stretched tight feeling it gives you, to hold the oxygen in. Now very slowly and purposefully, breathe out (through puckered lips), a long, steady exhale. Create an **image** in your mind to lengthen the exhale. For example, see yourself blowing the fuzzy seeds off of a dandelion that has gone to seed. Or, you are blowing a long steady note on a flute. Repeat this inhale holding it, followed with another slow, steady, long exhale. Determine during this inhalation and exhalation that these next few minutes belong only to you. Do not share them with anybody, or anything. Whatever problems, worries, or cares you have, including whatever it is you are going to do next in your day, briefly think what they are and list them all, by writing them on a mental chalkboard in your mind. Then, again mentally, take out a big chalk eraser and wipe each one off, one at a time, so that you are looking at an entirely blank slate, or chalkboard, in your mind. Verbalize a thought to yourself, like, "This is my time now (problem), and you are just going to have to wait." And then forget it during your relaxation technique!

2

Now follow your breathing cycle, whether it is fast, slow, regular, or irregular. Just mentally tune in and follow each inhale and each exhale. Picture yourself on an elevator, and each exhale is a ride down one more floor; each inhale is the brief pause for the floor stop, door opening and closing. Or, imagine that your mind is on a slow roller coaster ride of up and down, up and down.

3

As you begin to relax, you will experience that the exhalation (breathing out) becomes longer and longer. Don't interfere with your inhalation and exhalation— just ride with it and experience this longer ride out. This begins true relaxation.

4

At various times during the entire voluntary conscious relaxation technique, you will have to mentally tune back in to your breathing technique, for mastering this "roller coaster ride" is the **central focus** of your total control over relaxation.

Step 3: Tuning in to Various Parts of the Body

Let's start at the top of your head and travel down to the tips of your toes.

1

On the top of your head, mentally feel the "part" of your hair. Make it wide . . . just relax your scalp.

2

Mentally envision your ears. Drop all tension in your ears. If you are wearing earrings, mentally feel them on your earlobes.

3

Tune in to your forehead. Is it tense and full of wrinkles? Make it flat, and wide; no wrinkles; picture it smooth and shiny.

4

What is the space between your eyebrows doing? (Figure 7-3.) Is it grooved and full of wrinkles? Relax,

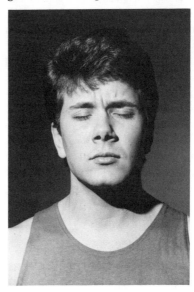

Figure 7-3.

with a wide space between your eyebrows. This is one of **the** telltale locations of human stress. A person who is highly stressed seems to permanently keep the space between the eyebrows tensed (contracted, wrinkled). Calm, serene people stand out by having this small space wide, relaxed, and untensed.

5

Relax your eyebrows as if heavy weights were pulling down the ends. This will also relax your temple area.

6

There is a hinge joint near your ear hole that is used to open and close your lower jaw. Relax that joint by dropping your lower jaw. It will make your lips part. Relax your chin.

7

When you relax your jaw, mentally feel your teeth and tongue. When some people try to practice total relaxation, they tightly press (tense) their tongue to the roof of their mouths. Also, many people grit or grind their teeth at night—an audible sign of tension in the area.

8

Relax your throat by thinking of the feeling you get with the second stage of swallowing. Persons who sing or play musical instruments have been trained in this technique to relax the area so that the best sounds will come out of a relaxed vocal mechanism.

9

Drop your shoulders and chest so that there is a wide space between your ears and shoulders. This is an area that we unconsciously tense throughout the day, unnecessarily. Whether we drive a car or walk in miserable weather, we tense the shoulders up near our ears and encourage neck aches and headaches. When you think about it next time, untense this group if you don't actually need to be holding it in a tensed manner.

10

Allow the weight of your chest to sink through to the floor. Think: heavy chest.

11

Drop all tension from your upper arms, elbows, lower arms, and hands until you can just feel your fingertips pulsating on the floor. A tingling feeling may be felt in your fingertips.

12

Relax your buttocks. This will hold the key in untensing the lower half of your body.

13

Relax your kneecaps. This joint connects your upper and lower leg, and many times we tense our knee area when we attempt to relax other body parts. When you relax the knees, the upper legs will relax, and the heavy weight of your legs will begin to drop to the floor. Likewise, the lower legs respond almost automatically, with the feet then rolling outward.

14

Mentally feel what your toes are doing in your shoes. Are they tensed and curled under? If so, relax them.

15

And now, return to the most difficult place to relax— the stomach and intestinal area. Focus your mind on the navel area and picture a wide, flat, picturesque pond. Envision a small pebble being tossed into the very center, with a soft, rippling effect occurring. Each ripple is a wave of relaxation. Feel the weight of your navel area sinking through, past your spine, onto the floor below you.

16

Now return back to your breathing cycle, and follow it several times. Remember to focus totally on the long, slow exhale.

17

Finally, retake a mental check of all body parts, beginning at the top part of your hair, traveling down to your toes, and finishing with your navel area.

18

Now just **rest** a few moments and enjoy the totally untensed feeling you are experiencing.

Step 4: Heart Rate Monitoring and Alert Stretch

1

In this lying down position, feel for your pulse. Mentally picture and feel your heart beating. Actively try to slow it down with your mind—cue it to beat slower.

2

Count your pulse for fifteen seconds and multiply by four for a minute heart rate count. How does this compare with your pre-activity heart rate count and your resting heart rate count? Isn't it phenomenal what three minutes of relaxation can do for your body's recovery from exercise?

3

You can now leave feeling totally renewed, refreshed, and in control of what remains of the rest of the day!

4

Before you get up, **sit up** slowly and stretch your arms, legs, chest, back, etc. so that you become alert immediately (Figure 7-4). You must do this fifteen-second stretch or you'll find yourself yawning for an hour afterward! Of course, if this relaxation procedure is practiced before going to bed, omit this "alert stretch."

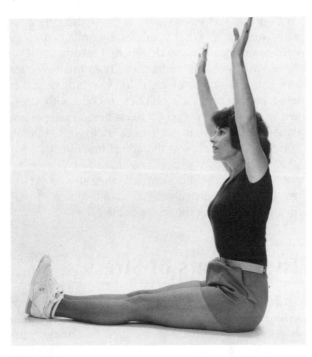

Figure 7-4.

The aforementioned steps were given in the form of mental cueing. Say and do each step **slowly** so that it takes on meaning. Perhaps you can tape your own voice, giving each cue slowly and playing it to yourself as you practice the skill of relaxation at home. It would be a lot easier than reading the cues to yourself and then trying to apply them during the relaxation.

When you have mastered this technique and developed total relaxation for yourself, you will find that you can apply this technique anywhere (with only slight changes in body position, etc.). **You can then incorporate this relaxation technique to all moments of stress** and develop total mental control. When you are in total control of your mind, in all circumstances, **no one** can bug you!

". . . imagery may well prove to be the single most important technique for modern health care."

—Jeanne Achterberg, Ph.D. and G. Frank Lawlis, Ph.D.[5]

There are many relaxation techniques that can help you find that inner stillness and peace that we all desire. Imaging is one that truly works if you will let it.

Stress Management

To fully understand how to manage the stress in your life, you must first understand what stress is and how you immediately react to it (both what bodily changes occur in you and what specific habits you rely upon to cope with it). You must then determine exactly what triggers the response recorded as "stressful" to you. You must finally get in concrete touch with a variety of positive techniques and skills that help you to adjust to the stressors you're encountering in life, and use them at a moment's notice! This will give you the total self-control you desire.

Understanding these four points are, briefly, how you learn to manage your stress. The remainder of this chapter will give you the information on point number one—what stress is, and on point number four—techniques and skills that help you to adjust.

To fully understand the second two points—how **you specifically react** to a variety of situations, and what type of stressors trigger you (set you off)—you must personally reflect upon and examine yourself. This self-assessment is found in the Appendix, Chart 9. Take an hour or so of "alone time," and complete this chart now. Try to imagine yourself using every reaction and situation presented, before you record what your response would be.

"To the possession of the self,
the way is inward."[6]

Just What Is Stress?

Probably the most noted scientific researcher in modern times on the topic of stress and its effect on the human body is the late Viennese-born endocrinologist, Hans Selye. He defines stress as the **nonspecific response of the body to any kind of demand that is made upon it.** From this definition you can now deduct that "stress" (at least scientifically described) is a neutral term. It can be **positive** (called "eustress") or **negative** (called "distress"). Finding, and being able to appreciate the balance between the two, is the challenge before you.

An analogy to more clearly understand the balance that must be established is this: stress is like the pressure in a tire. If there is no pressure, you won't be going anywhere. If the optimum amount (i.e., "balanced'') is present, you're going to have a smooth ride. If, however, too much pressure is present, you'll rockily bounce along and when there's an unexpected obstacle present or a weakness in it, it is going to blow out!

Or, it can be like the tension placed on a guitar string. If no tension is present, you'll have no sound. If the right amount is present, you can create a beautiful sound. But if too much tension is present, you'll either get an unacceptable sound you don't like to hear, or the string will snap!

Physiological Responses To Stress

The response your body exhibits to the positive or negative stressful demands that are made upon it from life situations includes the following:

- There is an increase of sugar in the blood.
- Your rate of breathing increases.
- Your heart rate increases.
- Your blood pressure increases.
- There is an activation of the blood clotting mechanism to protect you from injury.
- There is increased muscle tension.
- There is a cessation of digestion, and the blood is diverted to the brain and muscles.
- There is increased perspiration output.
- There is decreased salivation.
- There is a loosening of bladder and bowel muscles.
- There is an outpouring of various hormones, like adrenalin.
- Your pupils dilate.
- And there is a heightening of all of your senses.

In effect, then, your body goes into a ''RED ALERT'' and you are ready to fight or take off (flight). This has thus been named the ''fight or flight'' response to stress.

Many times you can't do either—fight or flight—and you must stay **in** the situation (and ''stew''). If this response (as characterized by the above list) is long enough or severe enough, you then experience wear and tear on your bodily systems. This leaves you open to the invasion of some sort of illness. It will **show up and affect the weakest link in your system first**, wherever that may be. For some it's one area (like a stomach ulcer) and for others, it's someplace else (like a heart attack).

Once a person becomes ill, then, illness also becomes a stressor. This will increase your stress response (again, as described in the list of bodily changes) and you may feel as if you are caught in a double-bind.[7]

Coping With Stress

In order to stay mentally balanced, we all do **something** to cope with the stress in our lives. Some of these coping mechanisms are positive and some of them are detrimental to our total well-being. Re-read the list of coping mechanisms called ''stress releases'' on Chart 9, and then note how **you** habitually cope with stress, i.e., what your positive means are and what your negative and detrimental means are.

You will probably come away from this reflection and self-assessment being a lot less judgmental of other people and their abilities to cope with stress. Just knowing that we all do **something** to relieve and cope with the stress in our lives can help you to tolerate another person's choices that sometimes directly affect you. You come away realizing that some people are not ''bad'' people (because, say, they smoke cigarettes) but are simply making a ''bad'' choice in their means of reducing the stress in their lives.

The Triggers of Stress

Life is experience and life is change. Many things in life can trigger the stress response in you. Something as simple as a fleeting thought can trigger this psychological response. A big step in understanding stress management is to realize that how you **think** about a life experience, a change, or a problem is more important than the actual experience, change, or problem itself.

What do you do when life hands you an unfair, dirty deal? Or, when you are greatly stressed by someone or something? Do you allow the situation to consume you? Or, do you dissect it, understand the underlying fear, anger, or other emotion that is present in it, and then **take an action** to overcome the situation?

For example, a teacher or a true friend can tell you that you need to gain some muscle weight in order to improve your well-being and not appear so sickly. You are grateful for their concern. But if someone you do not like tells you that you need to gain some weight so you don't look so sickly, you may be ready to ''go to the mats'' with them! How you **think** about a problem is the key.

When you are successful in **adjusting to and controlling your responses to stress**, it can provide you with growth and an increased confidence for meeting the next challenge (life situation) that comes to you.

For we each **learn** how to adjust to the everyday big and small problems and life situations that are presented to us on the stage of life. We are not "born" adjusted; we systematically learn adjustments. "Life is like climbing a slippery hill. You climb, you slip, you climb, you slip. **The measure of you as a person is: what do you do when you slip?**"[8] Educating ourselves on these aforementioned points is but one way to manage and adjust positively to our stress.

Management Techniques That Work

There are numerous techniques to incorporate in taking charge and action against stressors in life. Here are a few basic categories to consider:

- **Mental Skills:** imagery, self-hypnosis, relaxation techniques; thus the inclusion of this chapter of information in an "exercise" textbook.
- **Physical Skills:** exercising (aerobic dancing), massages, hug therapy.
- **Communication Skills:** using oral and body language to correctly inform your point of view, needs, wants, feelings.
- **Intellectual Skills:** philosophically defining parameters you can accept in human behavior; famous quotations to live by; religious ideas you follow.
- **Diversionary Techniques:** what you do in your free moments to positively distract you and release your stress—like hobbies and talents improvement.

A Final Thought

To manage your stress, you must **take time to look inward.** Developing your own physical and mental self to your fullest potential is an exciting life goal to set! It starts by providing yourself with **time** for a physical program, like aerobic dance, and continues during the final program moments of the aerobic dance hour with the relaxation phase. This conclusion is the mental "exercise" phase where **control is actively practiced** through imagery and relaxation techniques. Recognition, practice, and repetitions of all of your program techniques will help you in the management of stress in your life.

8

INDEPENDENCE!
Choreographing Your
Own Routines

To choreograph or plan your own routines, choose your favorite music with a moderate to fast tempo. Use songs that are upbeat and that give you a good feeling. Make sure that you will enjoy your choices, because you will be hearing them a lot—first as you choreograph and then as you dance. Remember that the dances you have learned and will be choreographing can be performed to different musical selections. Each dance doesn't have to be performed to the same song every time. The only exception is if you select to design the "advanced" choreography method with gestures and step patterns specifically planned to depict the mood and words to a particular song. The music that you select can be your best motivator to keep you dancing aerobically on a regular basis.

Guidelines for Choreographing

The following guidelines will help you choreograph your own routines:

1

Your dance does not need to last as long as the song.

2

You can choreograph one sequence and keep repeating it until the music is over. Two examples of this would be:

- A polka group dance, where everyone remains in contact in one large circle (arms on next person's close shoulder) and polkas together, using several varieties of polka steps, consisting of both various intensities and impacts.
- The "A-B-C-D" pattern repeated with the repetitions per foot that you design (i.e., left or right; 1's, 2's, 3's, or 4's).

3

You can choreograph two sequences and combine them in any way you want. For example, 1-2-1-2.

4

Make the dance sequence easy to learn and remember. If it becomes too complicated and you spend a lot of time learning it, you defeat the purposes of doing an aerobic dance—enjoyment and to keep moving without stopping.

5

As you create your dances, make sure that you sequence steps so you are moving continuously without any stopping from one movement to the next.

6

You can pace the routine by putting in low-impact steps like lunges, widestride varieties, walks, etc. that allow some "slowing down" or recovery, but not stopping. This is an especially useful technique for songs that last a long time. Of course, a dance of longer duration comes in your program after you've been aerobic dancing for at least six to nine sessions (a minimum of twenty minutes of aerobic dancing each session).

7

Keep your arms at or above your waist at all times. When you are first learning the footwork, you don't need to choreograph the arms yet. You do need to keep them in a jogger's position or at least above the waist. This helps keep the tension throughout the entire body and not just in the legs and feet.

8

As you develop your routine, use enough variety in step patterns and gesturing (arms, head, shoulders, hips, etc.) patterns to keep the dance interesting as well as challenging.

9

To determine if your dance is challenging enough (high-intensity level, fast tempo, and sufficient duration), check your pulse after doing the dance and see if you have reached your training zone.

10

If a particular step pattern or gesture is difficult to learn or remember, change it. You can always modify or change any part of your own dance or anyone else's to fit your own needs and abilities!

11

You have a repertoire of gestures and step patterns (see Chapter 5). Use these to begin, and then add your own creative moves. Chart 10 provides space to list and describe your creative new ideas.

12

Research professionals concerned with potential injuries have listed the following guidelines to consider and use when developing your own, or participating in, aerobic dance:

- To reduce the severity of impact shock on the lower extremities, repetitive jumping on the same foot should not exceed four consecutive jumps.
- Trunk rotation should be avoided while on the feet with hips or lower spine flexed. Rotational activity in this position subjects the intervertebral disks to very high mechanical stress.
- Extremes of joint flexion and extension (such as deep knee bends and ballistic hyperextension of the knee) should be avoided. Such movements can expose connective tissues around joints to ex-

tremely high mechanical stresses.
- The feet should be moved repeatedly to prevent cramping in the intrinsic muscles of the foot.[1]

13

As the tempo of your music increases your dance steps to a faster tempo, you need to take smaller steps and use less space. This enables you to stay with the beat of the music. For example, you do a slide and you cover three feet of space with each slide. As you put the slide to fast music, you only have time enough to cover one foot of space. Your slide will need to be smaller to fit the music and to allow you to keep on the beat.

14

Be sure that you determine the underlying or steady beat of the music. (This can be accomplished by clapping or writing down each beat.) This will determine how easy you will be able to choreograph and perform to it. Count the underlying beats in sets of eight. (Most music that you'll choose will be in 4/4 time to make this counting possible.)

15

If you have difficulty with tempo or phrasing or in finding the underlying beat, it would be best to find another song or version of the same song.

16

Choreograph to the set of eight beats rather than to the melody, for "easy" or "moderate" difficulty dances (see Chart 10 in the Appendix). The only times that the melody or overlying beat is important to choreographing is when it repeats itself and you wish to do the same step sequence each time, i.e., each time the **chorus** is repeated in the song, or you are "advanced" choreographing to the mood and words of a particular song.

17

After you have determined your step patterns, decide how many times you will repeat the step pattern. Repeat the same step patterns two, four, eight, or sixteen times. You want to repeat just enough to make the dance easy to remember. However, if you have too many repetitions it will become boring to dance.

18

Start each new step sequence with the right foot to make the transition smoother. Very seldom do you need to start with the left foot. You want the transitions smooth and continuous so that your pulse rate stays in your training zone.

19

After writing the step sequences down on paper, mentally go through the dance as you listen to the music.

20

Once you have the step patterns sequenced and are able to coordinate them with the music, then coordinate and add the arms, or other gestures, with your steps. "Gestures" are defined as the movement of any non-weight-bearing body part.

21

Progression from "easy" to "advanced" choreography is your ultimate goal. Begin with a dance using basic "easy" steps. As you are able to accomplish this, move on to a "moderate difficulty" by combining coordination-combination moves, with several easy basic transitional moves included. When you desire a most difficult challenge, try choreographing easy to difficult step and gesture patterns to a particular song that you wish to interpret (mood and/or words). This is where aerobic dance bridges the gap between just exercise dance and performance dance. This gives a challenge to those individuals who are needing and wanting their aerobic dance experience to also fulfill their desire to express themselves aesthetically! And this is how individualized programming is accomplished.

22

Remember you are choreographing a fitness dance, so be sure that you execute the steps and gestures with tension (firmness) throughout your body and that your spine is always stabilized, using good body position throughout. A relaxed, easy style won't overload the heart enough to give you the proper training zone workout and may encourage dynamically poor body positioning (poor posture while moving through space).

23

Chart 10 in the Appendix provides several samples of choreographed dances from easy, moderately difficult, to advanced to fit your individualized needs. Attempt the planned dances and follow with developing your own. **Enjoy your independence!**

Suggestions for Movement Patterns

Suggestions for movement patterns that will help you choreograph routines are as follows:

Locomotor Activities

Movement that carries the body from one place to another through space.

- Galloping
- Hopping
- Jumping
- Jogging
- Leaping
- Marching
- Prancing
- Rocking
- Running
- Skipping
- Sliding
- Strutting
- Walking

Jumping: There are five basic "jumps." They are:

Take-off	Landing

One foot to the same foot (also called a hop).
One foot to the other foot (called a leap).
One foot to two feet (called a stride).
Two feet to two feet (close or widestride).
Two feet to one foot (called a hopscotch).

Non-Locomotor Activities

Movement performed over a stationary base, of low impact:

- Bending
- Bouncing
- Closing
- Curling
- Gesturing
- Kicking (from the ankle, knee, hip)
- Lunging
- Opening
- Pulling
- Pushing
- Shaking
- Stretching
- Swaying
- Swinging (arms, legs, torso)
- Turning
- Twisting

Body Shapes

- Straight or angular
- Widespread
- Round
- Twisted
- Symmetrical
- Asymmetrical

Directionality

- Up
- Down
- Right side
- Left side
- Forward
- Back
- Diagonal

Force

- Light
- Heavy
- Gradually
- Suddenly

Speed

- Fast
- Slow
- Gradually
- Suddenly

Pathways

- Curved (i.e., circle, figure 8)
- Straight
- Combinations of straight and curved
- Diagonals (i.e., zig zags)

Levels
(of the body as well as different body parts)

- Low
- Medium
- High

Extensions of Different Body Parts

- Elbows
- Arms
- Hands
- Legs
- Upper torso

Dance Steps

- Polka
- Charleston
- Cha-cha
- Grapevine
- Hustle
- Two-step
- Jitterbug
- Disco step
- Foxtrot

Dances

- Mexican hat dance
- Bunny hop (an American line dance)
- Hora (Israeli folk dance)
- Square dancing

Adding Sound To Movement

- Clap
- Slap (knees, thighs)
- Click fingers
- Audibles (u-u-u-h!)

Adding Creativity to Movement

Allow the creative right half of your brain to kick into action. Here are several creative ideas to start the gears moving:

- Create the alphabet from A to Z with your body, using any of the former suggestions (i.e., locomotor the letter over the floor space; non-locomotor the letter—Figure 8-1, a stretching widestride letter **M**; or body-shape the letter—Figure 8-2, a standing letter **K**.

Figure 8-1.   **Figure 8-2.**

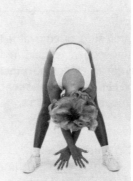 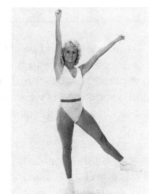

- Create your phone number using step and gesture patterns.
- Write a brief message to someone you miss.

Now list your new creative ideas on Chart 10 in the Appendix. Creativity and variety eliminate boredom!

Combining Steps and Beats

As you begin choreographing your aerobic dances, keep the steps simple. First, try four steps and keep repeating them. For example:

- **Jog**, 16 times   16 counts
- **Hop, kick**, four times   8 counts
- **Rock**, 4 times   8 counts   **40 counts**
- **Jump, circling**, 4 times   8 counts

You have a forty-count sequence that you can keep repeating throughout the song you have chosen.
Put these steps with your **underlying beats.**

/   /   /   /   /   /   /   /   = 8 beats

Jog each beat = 8 times

/   /   /   /   /   /   /   /   = 8 beats
Jog each beat = 8 times

/   /   /   /   /   /   /   /   = 8 beats
Hop kick (takes 2 beats at a time) = 4 times

/   /   /   /   /   /   /   /   = 8 beats
Rock (1 beat forward, 1 beat backward for each rock) = 4 times

/   /   /   /   /   /   /   /   = 8 beats
Jump circling (two-foot jump takes 1 beat, hold and clap takes 1 beat) = 4 times

Now it wouldn't be very interesting or enjoyable to keep repeating this forty-count sequence standing in one place, so look at the different aspects of movement and decide ways in which you can make the sequence more fun and challenging to learn and perform.
For example:

- Jog, 8 times forward; jog, 8 times backward.
- Hop and kick diagonally alternating feet, 4 times (i.e., hop right, kick left leg to diagonal right; hop

left, kick right leg to diagonal left).
- Rock forward and backward 2 times; rock right side to left side 2 times.
- Jump and hold turning right, completing a circle; or jump and hold turning left, completing a circle.

Now add a variety of gestures to your sequence:

- Jog with arms at side (above the waist) using jogger's arms, or, like window-wiper blades.
- Hop kick with arms shoulder height and straight ahead; or out to the sides.
- Rock with arms in same position as in the hop kick; or add finger clicking.
- Jump with arms raised straight above your shoulders; or add a clap in front of your chest.

Pull all this together with your music and enjoy! As you begin to feel comfortable with your choreographing, add more basic steps and coordination patterns to your sequence to increase the challenge. The next progression would be to plan two or more different sequences for a more interesting and challenging dance. Progression is systematical. As you understand, attempt more.

Independence Day!

You will not need for someone else to plan your movements—you now have learned the basic index variety of possibilities, have created new possibilities of your own, and have the know-how to combine and plan, i.e., "choreograph" all of your own aerobic dance routines. With your favorite music and your enjoyable, vigorous routines, you're on your way to developing your own aerobic dance program.

9

UNDERSTANDING YOUR BODY TYPE, BODY COMPOSITION, AND WEIGHT CONTROL

"You have to spend every minute of your life in your own company.
If you don't enjoy it, you're going to be miserable."
Dr. Normal Vincent Peale
Positive Imaging

When asked why they are taking a fitness course, nine out of ten persons have responded "to improve my figure/physique by toning muscles and losing weight."[1] A simple yet concrete goal. We seem to readily admit to the fact that a primary goal is to **appear** healthy and slim—to either ourselves or to others.

Why do individuals today desire this goal? It's because we can directly see when our body looks nice, lean, and toned; likewise, we can directly see when it looks out of shape, flabby, and full of fat deposits. When it comes to improvement, many individuals will therefore initially focus on this **concrete** form of their understanding of "fitness" or "being in shape"— that which they can directly **see**.

Your outer appearance is not, however, the entire (or even major) focus of a quality fitness program. Chapter 1 mentioned that you can live without well-toned muscles or a trim figure, but you can't live long without a good strong heart and lungs. However, it is difficult to have "life-sustaining" goals such as heart and lung fitness uppermost in mind, because you just

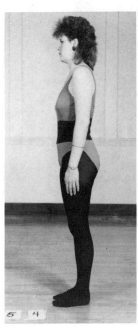 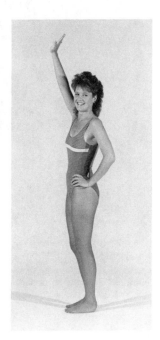

Figure 9-1.   **Figure 9-2.**

can't **see** your heart, lungs, or blood vessels. Therefore, acknowledging and understanding the accompanying facets and the admitted personal priorities that people bring to a fitness program is indeed necessary. **Looking attractive and feeling good about and accepting your appearance** are important ancillary goals to have and understand. Since you can directly and concretely **see** and experience this quality, and admit to this being a top priority anyway, let's size up what each of us has to "work with" and set some attainable goals.

Realistic Self-Appraisal

To understand what your best outer physical appearance can be, you must first recognize and **accept** your very makeup. At conception we were all blessed with a specific genetic makeup for which we can thank our parents! We each possess a specific body type (physical classification of the human body), and we can never be the size and shape of someone whom we idolize—be that person smaller or bigger than we are!

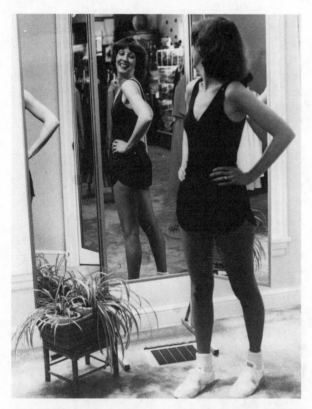

Figure 9-3. In order to understand what our best outer physical appearance can be, we must first recognize and accept our very makeup.

Sheldon[2] differentiates between body types and accompanying characteristics (extremes) as follows. Which do you seem to be most like?

Endomorphy—roundness and softness of the body. Features of this type:

- Short neck.
- High square shoulders.
- Large abdomen over thorax.
- Breasts developed.
- Round full buttocks.
- Skin is soft and smooth.

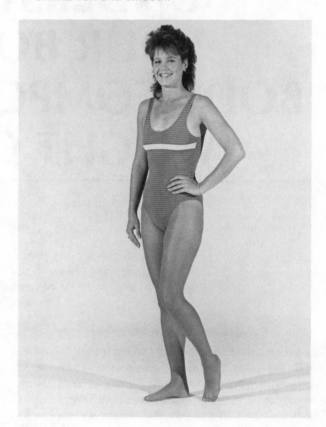

Figure 9-4.

Mesomorphy—square body with hard, rugged, prominent muscles. Features:

- Large bones covered with thick muscle.
- Forearm thickness; heavy wrists, hands, and fingers.
- Slender waist.
- Broad shoulders.
- Trunk upright.

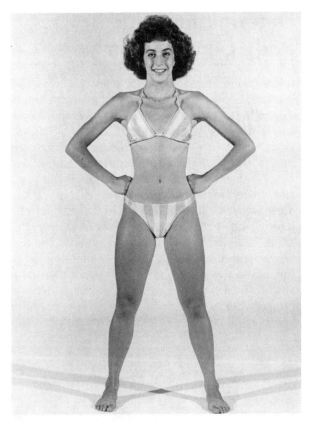

Figure 9-5.

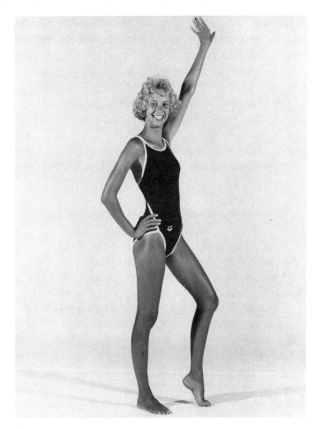

Figure 9-6.

Ectomorphy—linearity, fragility, and delicacy of body. Features:

- Small bones.
- Thin muscles.
- Shoulders droop; not much muscularity.
- Long limbs and short trunk (not necessarily a tall person, though).
- No bulging muscles anywhere.
- Shoulder blades tend to wing out in back.

Once you begin to realize that you have a specific body type, you can begin to understand a second component of the self-appraisal. This is understanding what makes up your body mass, or "body composition."

Understanding Body Composition

Your body is composed of two weights: **lean weight** and **fat weight**. Lean weight is composed of your bones, muscles, and internal organs. Fat weight is just that. It is the stored energy that you are wearing for

future use. The amount of each that you carry is important to know to understand what is best for the health of your heart and lungs (i.e., "cardiorespiratory" system).

Your lean weight declines (weighs less) after maturity (when you stop growing) at a certain steady pace every year. This is one of the beautiful aging processes. To slow down the aging processes and maintain your strength, you need to incorporate muscular strength and endurance (explained in Chapter 6) as part of your total fitness program. Basically, the only portion of your lean weight that you can greatly change (for the better) is your muscle weight. It's rather difficult to increase lean weight by making your bones heavier or by increasing the size of your liver! (Remember— lean weight equals bones, muscles, and internal organs.) You can, however, increase your lean weight through a muscle-thickening program called strength training or weight training. Since thicker (denser) muscle fiber weighs more, your lean weight will increase.

For each individual's amount of lean, a certain percentage of fat can be "worn" to maintain ideal cardiorespiratory efficiency. Body fat has several necessary functions:

1

To provide storage for the fat-soluble vitamins A, D,

E, and K. (The other vitamins are water-soluble, and if they are not used daily as taken in, they are excreted through the urine, etc.)

2

To insulate the body from the weather.

3

To protect the internal organs from shocks and blows delivered to the body, i.e., falls, physical contact, etc.

4

To provide the storage of future energy (go-power).

Beyond supplying these needs, you just don't need the extra weight and stress that fat places on the heart.

An appropriate percentage of fat to be worn with the lean is approximately 20 to 22 percent body fat for women and 10 to 12 and one-half percent body fat for men. Women carry a higher percentage of fat because an extra layer of fat is present below the skin and because breast tissue is primarily fat. But if you wear more fat tissue than the suggested amounts, it simply adds additional risk factors associated with heart disease. If you wear **less** than the above ideal percentage, it doesn't matter UNLESS:

- You are malnourishing yourself.
- You cosmetically wish to look heavier.

For instance, endurance athletes (like marathon runners or Olympic gymnasts) do not carry the suggested ideal percentage. They carry much less. They simply burn it off and don't carry the excess. They (usually) eat right to provide the necessary nutrients and energy and thus display a firm, trim, toned look. The wobbly-fat, "gelatin" look is absent from these extremely physical people, and yet they stay well.

In contrast are the anorexic individuals (persons who exhibit the starvation disease, anorexia nervosa). They also may carry less than the suggested ideal percentage of body fat and accomplish this feat through a process of **also eliminating their lean weight**. They desire a trim look but go about it in a way that is against all physiological principles of proper weight loss. To them, weight loss means purely **dropping pounds** to be slim at all costs, no matter what kind of weight it is, fat **or** lean. This is an extremely detrimental way to lose weight!

To enable individuals to understand healthy slimness and unhealthy slimness, an indepth look at weight control follows later in this chapter.

Determining Your Body Composition

You cannot determine the amount of body fat and lean that a person has merely by looking at him/her (Figure 9-7). An assessment of body composition involves determining as precisely as possible an individual's body fat and lean body weight. Such an assessment allows an **accurate estimate** to be made of what an individual's ideal weight should be. This is important, since the traditional approach of using standardized weight tables adjusted for sex, height, and frame size has been shown to be grossly inaccurate for a rather large percentage of the population. The ideal weight within any one category of these tables can vary up to twenty-two pounds. It is not unusual for an individual to fall within the normal range for his/her category but to actually have ten to thirty pounds of excess body fat.[4]

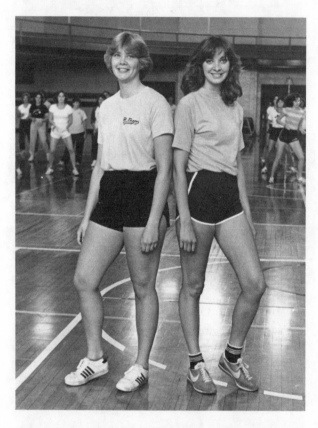

Figure 9-7. It is impossible to determine "ideal weight" just by looking at someone. Both of these college women are approximately 5'10" tall and are carrying the same percentage of body fat (28%) on their individual leans. At left, Paula's ideal weight is 145. On the right, Jill's ideal weight is 114.

Consequently, measurement techniques have been sought to more accurately determine whether an individual is overweight (overfat) or obese and then quantify exactly by how much. Several excellent techniques are available:

- Measuring skinfold thickness.
- Analysis by electrical impedance.
- Underwater weighing (specific gravity).
- Using both skinfold thickness and anthropometric measures of bone thickness and/or girth measurements.

Because of ease of use in an aerobic dance setting and availability of equipment, only the first technique will be fully detailed here. However, analysis by electrical impedance and underwater weighing (specific gravity) will be covered briefly.

Measuring Skinfold Thickness

There are a number of skinfold measurement formulas that use various sites on the body for calculations. A formula that is preferred to be used for aerobic dance class purposes was developed by Dr. Jack H. Wilmore, then of the University of California at Davis. According to Wilmore,[5] lean body weight, percentage of fat, and relative weights for an individual can be accurately measured by the following formula, which has a coefficient of correlation of .90 to .95 r. In mathematical terminology, this means that it is a quite accurate measurement tool for persons aged eighteen through thirty-five who are not extremely obese. The three steps to this procedure are as follows. Chart 11 in the Appendix is provided to help you determine you body composition, and to provide you with a **concrete** method of setting your weight goals.

1
Step 1 determines how much lean weight (bones, muscles, and organs) you have, **in pounds.**

2
Step 2 determines the **percentage** of fat that you are carrying along with your lean weight. You can thus place yourself in a category of relative percent fat (the ratio of fat to fat-free weight). The four categories described here are ''obesity,'' ''overweight,'' ''ideal weight,'' and ''underfat weight.''

3
Step 3, then, determines **relative weights for you** by

giving you your pound weights (when you step on a scale) for the four categories described. You are then able to realize how much fat weight, in pounds, you need to lose, gain, or maintain to be at the ideal percentage of fat to lean, and therefore at your **ideal weight**. It thus gives you concrete numbers with which to set goals. Rather than the abstract thought, ''I think I need to lose twenty-five pounds,'' you can say with assurance to yourself, ''I need to lose eighteen to twenty-one pounds of body fat at my present lean weight.''

Ongoing, Lifetime Assessment

To initiate this procedure today, or at any future date, an individual needs only to have access to two accurate measurement tools:

- A ''doctor's'' scale to determine the present accurate nude weight, in pounds.
- A calibrated, precision instrument called a ''skinfold caliper,'' which will determine the present skinfold thickness, in millimeters. (Incidentally, the inexpensive plastic-type devices available are about as accurate as using your index finger, thumb, and a ruler, and pinching an inch!) You are interested in **accuracy**, so use a precision instrument made by a reputable company.

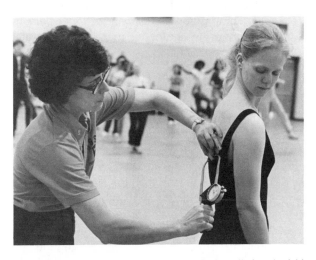

Figure 9-8. A calibrated, precision instrument called a skinfold caliper determines the present skinfold thickness, in millimeters. Measurement is taken subscapular in women.

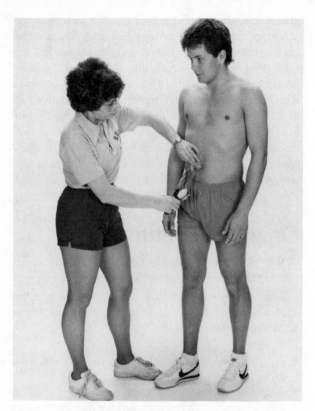

Figure 9-9. Measurement is taken vertically to the side of the navel in men.

Underwater Weighing

After middle age, body density changes, and the skinfold measurement procedure becomes a less accurate tool, especially for inactive people. A more accurate body composition assessment for older persons (or for persons of any age for that matter) is underwater weighing.

This technique requires a special facility with a water tank and a submersible scale upon which the individual sits. Specific gravity is determined (ratio of the density of the person to the density of the water). Since an object immersed in a fluid loses an amount of water equivalent to the weight of the fluid that is displaced[6], and since the density of the object is two and one-half times greater than the density of water,[7] an individual's specific gravity can be determined. A figure can then be calculated to represent the percentage of fat. All of the above configurations tell an individual the correct amount of lean weight, the percentage of fat currently present, and the ideal weight toward which the individual should work (if not presently there).

Analysis of Total Body Water by Electrical Impedance

Electrical impedance has been used in the laboratory for over forty years. Its applications to the estimation of total body water was successfully done in the 1970s. In the late 1970s and early 1980s the application of the technique was perfected for measuring lean body mass. (This methodology became commercially available in 1982.)

Bioelectrical impedance measurement of total body water (and thus body fat) is accomplished by using a computer-like analyzer. Electrodes are placed on the right hand and right foot while the subject is lying down. A harmless current is transmitted from electrode to electrode at 800 microamps.

The resistance to the electrical current, instantaneously measured by the analyzer, is related to the total body water. Lean body mass is then calculated from knowing total body water. Body fat is determined by subtraction (i.e., total body water minus lean body mass equals body fat present).[8]

It is recommended that this resistance measurement be made before exercise, and at least three hours after eating, with no alcohol consumption for the forty-eight hours prior to the analysis. This measurement is very sensitive to diuretic medication (which promotes the excretion of urine) and other conditions which affect body water and electrolyte balance. Accurate results will not likely be obtained if these variables are present.

Bioelectrical impedance measurement is fast and takes less than three minutes, start to finish, including placement of the two electrodes. It is FDA approved, with no known contra-indications and is safe for individuals of all ages, in all conditions, including pregnancy, heart conditions (or with pacemakers present), or in the presence of orthopedic metals.[9]

Its accuracy is relative to underwater (hydrostatic) weighing and has been used in various research settings. With this analysis you receive a two-page computer printout of individualized information which includes the following: percentage of body fat, the actual weight of your fat pounds, lean body weight, total body water, your recommended weight, fat pounds to lose, a personalized weight loss chart (if you need to lose), your estimated basal metabolism, an individualized caloric expenditure chart detailing approximately a dozen different activities, and general exercise recommendations to enable you to obtain/maintain good health. When a significant change has been experienced in the amount of lean weight or fat weight present, an individual is then encouraged to be re-analyzed.

What Do the Fat % Age Categories Mean?

Visually, in terms of a traffic light, "obesity" is the red light—STOP NOW and think what all this extra fat is doing to your cardiorespiratory health. "Obesity" describes when a woman is 30 percent (or more) body fat and a man is 20 percent (or more) body fat to the amount of lean they are carrying. If lean weight increases (due to a weight training program, etc.), the percentage of fat worn with that lean will go up, i.e., your ideal weight would go up. But since your lean weight **declines** as you age, your ideal weight declines because you want to wear still 20 to 22 percent fat (women) or 10 to 12 and one-half percent fat (men) on that declining lean. Therefore, your ideal weight usually decreases with age. If you remain the same weight as when you were first married thirty years ago, you have usually gained extra **fat** weight. Because your activity level and metabolism both slow down with age, increasing your exercise and decreasing your food intake will assist you with your ongoing lifetime assessment process.

"Overweight" is the yellow light, "caution" category. Beware! You are in the category where many Americans are finding themselves today—creeping overfatness. Since you are "overfat," you need to be aware of your intake and output of energy (eating and exercising). For women, it's 25 to 29 percent body fat, and for men it's 15 to 19 percent body fat.

"Ideal weight" is the "go-for-it" three-pound range of your current lean weight wearing a specific proper percentage of fat. For women it is 20 to 22 percent fat, and for men it's 10 to 12 and one-half percent fat. Your ideal weight changes in proportion to your lean weight change(s).

"Underfat" depicts the individual who is carrying less than the suggested ideal percentage of body fat to the amount of lean that she/he has. Again, it doesn't matter how underfat you are as long as you eat right and don't malnourish your body.

With the aforementioned formula (and there are other excellent ones to use), you can, on a continual, lifetime basis, assess the ideal weight for your heart's best health.

Weight Control

Weight control equals controlling the amount of body fat that you carry in relation to the amount of lean you have. The principles of weight control include all of the following: **weight maintenance** (staying the same composition of fat to the amount of lean that you're carrying), **weight gain** (almost always in terms of lean weight gain, not fat weight gain), and **weight loss** (always in terms of loss of body fat).

Weight Maintenance

This refers to the fact that:

- Your current composition of fat to lean is ideal for your best cardiorespiratory health.
- You are pleased with how you look (cosmetically). You have enough strength to function well in your daily life of work and recreation, to whatever extreme that may encompass. To remain at this constant weight, your **energy** must be in balance, i.e.:

"calories in" = "calories out"
(eating) = (expenditure; exercise)

Since a decline in "calories out" occurs with aging (your metabolism slows down and you are less active), a decline in "calories in" (eat less) must accompany the aging processes.

Weight Gain

This almost always refers to the gaining of lean tissue, or the thickening of muscle fiber. When you want to cosmetically look better, or to have an increased amount of strength for a sport or for daily needs, weight training is the type of activity in which to engage. Since you would be using more energy in a day than you did prior to the weight training program, you would need to "calories in" (eat) the **same** amount as you are newly expending (in the form of "calories out") with weight training, for maintenance. However, to **gain lean** and **lose extra body fat** simultaneously requires you to **eat less** while providing the **increased exercise** of weight training. Only if you are at ideal weight or underfat weight should you accompany this weight-gain program with an increase in caloric intake.[10]

Weight gain would then directly mean an increase in muscle mass, or thickening those "rubber bands" that you have as muscles! Thicker rubber bands (i.e., muscles) are more dense and weigh more than thin rubber bands. You primarily do not gain more muscle cells—you thicken what you presently have.

Weight Loss

This always refers to the purposeful losing of **fat**

weight—never lean weight. Weight loss, of course, can occur to both your lean and your fat, according to how you go about losing the weight. The director of the local Better Business Bureau has stated that one of the top two frauds with which he comes in contact involves weight loss products and information.

"People will do anything to lose weight. You would be amazed at the amount of fraud that is being perpetrated on the American public. If it's easy, people will try it! If you want to get rich quick, go into the weight loss business."[11] This last statement was, of course, spoken in jest, but is, sadly, very true. Before you spend your money on any claim, product, device, or book, call your local Better Business Bureau. However, if you understand the principles of weight loss, you will always be able to determine a product's (program's, etc.) worth before you spend time, money, and energy on it.

A Case Study on Weight-Loss Product Use

A student who had been skinfold tested at the onset of a ten-week fitness course requested input on a weight-loss product that she was planning to use. The label stated that the product was to be consumed three times a day for one month. No other food was to be taken in. (The product is a powder in a can and is to be mixed with liquid.) It provides all the nutrients needed daily. It is recommended that exercise not accompany the use of the product. At the end of one month, when you have lost a substantial amount of weight, you eat regular meals again. Five pages of accompanying research (that comes with the product) **state that the product will cause you to lose only fat weight and not lean,** and quotes by various physicians worldwide claim the product's authenticity.

After much discussion with both a resident physiologist and a nutrition specialist who attempted to encourage the student against the product's use, the student still took the powder. Approximately three **weeks later, the student said that she had lost twelve** pounds and requested a second skinfold test. Of the twelve pounds of weight loss, **eight pounds were lean** and four were fat! She was totally crushed that this new "miracle" product was assisting her in losing primarily her lean weight—rapidly.

A key lesson was learned early in life for this nineteen-year-old woman. Not only did she lose a substantial amount of lean weight, but when she begins to eat normally again, she will more than likely gain weight, **all of which will be fat** (if no strength training is incorporated).

Principles of Weight Loss (i.e., Fat Loss)

1
Fat weight is the only kind of weight to lose. When a product claims to "get rid of excess body fluids," beware! Body fluids are not fat! (Incidentally, unnatural water retention, or edema, is a condition to be monitored and treated by a doctor, not by your self-prescribed procedures or products.)

2
If you lose water weight (fluids) by sweating during exercise, you will, and should, gain it back in twenty-four hours to maintain your body's beautifully synchronized chemical balance. The energy-producing (metabolic) processes perform best when all of the necessary components are present. So don't be misled into believing that dropping your water weight is effective weight loss. It is part of your fat-free weight and is a vital part of your continuous well-being. You can understand, then, why weighing yourself **after** a strenuous exercise session is an inaccurate time to weigh.

3
Fat is metabolized more readily and efficiently by performing high- or low-intensity exercise for a long duration of time. If you are fit to work at high intensity (i.e., at the upper end of your training zone—fully explained in Chapter 2) for over thirty minutes, you will have provided yourself with the most physiologically sound way to metabolize (burn off) that unwanted body fat.

Endurance exercise depends on fuel being furnished to the muscles, and liquid fat—cholesterol and triglycerides—is a far more important fuel than carbohydrates. Any exercise that lasts longer than thirty minutes must be nourished by liquid fat. Muscles burn fat directly—scientists thought that carbohydrates were the main fuel. That's only partially true. Carbohydrates are quickly exhausted. After fifteen minutes of exercise, fat is burning, and after thirty minutes, the nutrition is almost wholly fat—the same fat that has been clogging the arteries of the cardiovascular system.[12]

The conclusion of one research study at the University of Illinois is that **you need to exercise for MORE than THIRTY MINUTES at a time to make significant changes in the FAT content of the body.**

Wearing rubber suits, see-through plastic wrap around body parts, and on hot days heavy, long-sleeved "sweats," nylons, or tights will tend to inhibit the free flow of sweat and will disallow it to perform **its function of cooling you.** When it is hot and humid, wear as little as possible when performing fitness exercises. You cannot metabolize (burn up) fat faster by increasing your body temperature through the wearing of more clothes!

4

Fat will metabolize off your body in a general way. You can't "spot reduce!" Spot reducing is perhaps the most prevalent misconception concerning fat weight loss and the one by which many unscrupulous people are defrauding unsuspecting overfat Americans out of millions of dollars every year.

By your genetic constitution, your body will use up its stored energy (fat) any way in which it is programmed to do so. You cannot do fifty leg lifts a day and hope to reduce the fat deposits in that area. You will shape up (thicken) the muscle fiber in the area, and toned muscles contain more of the enzymes involved in breaking down fat—but you do not burn off the fat there, or at any one particular location, necessarily. As energy is needed, it is withdrawn—first from the immediate sources—and when this is used up, it is withdrawn randomly from more permanent storage. It is then converted to an immediate usable form. Thus, you may lose weight in places you don't necessarily wish to at first, like your face, chest, breast area, etc. But with a little perseverance, you'll metabolize off the fat in problem areas, too.

5

Fat weight loss is most readily accomplished through a combined program of dieting and exercising. It is very difficult to lose fat weight by only exercising more, and not changing your eating habits (less "calories in"). And when you **only diet** (eat less food) and step on a scale, the weight loss is not all fat! According to the way in which you have dieted, your weight loss is approximately one-half to two-thirds (50 to 68 percent) fat loss and one-third to one-half (33 to 50 percent) lean weight loss. And if your lifestyle and habits of eating and exercising don't change, after you stop dieting and you gain back your lost weight, **what you gain back is all fat.** You are therefore worse off! You lost both fat and lean and regained back only fat. Over a lifetime of this "yo-yo" crash dieting, you can see how you are detrimentally changing your entire body composition.

When you diet (eat less) and exercise (expend more calories or energy), you tend to lose approximately 100 percent fat. This is the only kind of weight that you want to lose. And exercise speeds weight loss, not only by burning calories while you're working out, but also by revitalizing your metabolism so that you **continue** to burn calories more readily for the next few hours.

6

You can both gain weight and lose weight with an endurance exercise program. You will be metabolizing off fat for energy (loss) and building up muscle (gain) simultaneously. So if you do not realize a change on the scale immediately, don't be disappointed!

7

A light exercise program will increase your appetite, and a strenuous exercise program will decrease your appetite. You will especially find that after an endurance (aerobic) hour, your desire for food greatly diminishes. You will have time to carefully select, or prepare, what you know is good for you, rather than ravenously grab that easy, high-calorie junk food just sitting around.

8

It is easier to eat less food than it is to exercise it off. Consider the following for a 120- 130-pound person:

- It takes approximately two minutes to walk off (two steps per second) one potato chip (ten calories).
- It takes five minutes of high-intensity aerobic dancing (eight calories per minute times five equals forty calories) to a fast-tempoed song to dance off one-sixth of a candy bar that contains 240 calories; i.e., one bite equals five minutes!
- In most high-intensity fitness sessions, you will only burn about 300 calories. So think twice about rewarding yourself with high-calorie treats afterward if you are seriously interested in losing your extra fat weight. Instead, replenish your water loss with no-calorie, yet quite filling, ice water.

9

Since there is no such thing as a constipated endurance aerobic dancer/athlete, you will, with regularity, eliminate your solid wastes. Regular, rhythmic stimulation of the entire digestion and elimination processes will be one of the side benefits that you'll not necessarily talk about, but for which you will certainly be glad!

10

The basic, bottom-line principle for fat weight loss is: the body's ENERGY BALANCE determines whether or not a person gains or loses body fat. Two words— ENERGY BALANCE—how very simple it all is. And yet look at all of the products, devices, and books that people buy to find the magic easy way. There simply is no magic—just **self-discipline** to understand that energy is the basis for change and will result in a proper weight loss if less caloric energy is intaken and more caloric energy is expended.

Caloric Intake and Use

Everything that you eat or drink becomes "you" for either a short or lengthy duration of time. Thus, you are what you eat! This means that the food nutrients you eat are used to maintain basic body functions such as breathing, blood circulation, normal body temperature, and growth and repair of all tissue and are related to fixed factors such as age, body size, and physiological state. Any kind of caloric intake that your body doesn't use or doesn't eliminate through solid or liquid waste is kept and "worn" as body fat for future energy needs. Thus, if you don't use it, or eliminate it, you **wear** it!

Caloric Expenditure

Every moment of every day, no matter what activity you are engaged in—from sleeping to aerobically dancing—you are using up calories. **Caloric energy expenditure is most influenced by your lifestyle— how physically active you are all day. The body's basic needs are more or less fixed, but the amount of physical exertion in which you engage is a personal decision.**

How physically active your life is depends on choice of profession (a fitness instructor usually has more opportunities for vigorous physical exercise than a school bus driver or a college dean) and choice of recreational activities (playing cards requires fewer calories than leisurely walking).

It all depends upon a multitude of day-to-day choices: whether to walk to the local store or drive the car; use the stairs or elevator; rake the leaves or hire it done; go out for a bicycle ride after supper or watch a TV show. **How physically active your life is depends as much on attitude as it does on opportunity.**[13]

Formula For Weight Maintenance

If you can image a picture of "energy in" and "energy out" balanced, you can then understand maintenance, or staying the same weight. To remain at the same weight, you must intake (eat) the amount of calories you expend (burn up) every day.

How much energy you eat and expend every day to stay at your current weight is determined next:

Figuring Weight Maintenance

A. Record your present weight, in pounds: _____

B. Record your type of life-style; number values are: ___
   12—sedentary
   15—active physically
   18—pregnant/nursing
   20—varsity athlete or physical laborer

C. Multiply A times B: _____
This is your weight maintenance number, or the **number of calories per day you now eat to stay at your current weight.**

Caloric Expenditure for Various Activities

How many calories you burn per minute during any activity depends upon two criteria:

- The **intensity** at which you perform the exertion (high-, medium-, or low-level work or exercise— i.e., run, jog, walk).
- Your body weight.

The higher the intensity, the more calories you burn per minute. (You expend more energy and calories running a mile than you do walking that mile.) And the heavier you are, the more calories per minute you will burn. (Full-sized cars burn more fuel per mile than the small compact models.)

For an understanding of your own daily caloric expenditure, turn to Chart 15 in the Appendix. By using the list of various activities and intensities, and figuring how many calories you burn per minute per kilogram of your body weight, then enumerating how many minutes you performed the exertion on one day, and then adding up all your "energy out" activities, you arrive at a figure which totals **your caloric expenditure for that one day.**

If it is close to the same number of calories you intake (eat) in one day (just established above), you will remain at your current weight. That is weight maintenance for you.

Caloric Intake Needed To Gain Lean Weight

The caloric requirement to add one pound of body

muscle is 2,500 calories. (This includes about 600 calories for the "muscle," and the extra energy needed for exercise to develop the muscle.) Thus, the **daily caloric excess, over your maintenance number just figured, is 360 calories.**[14]

You must first, however, be at or below your ideal weight to go on an excess calorie eating program to gain muscle. You want to use your excess body fat first for your energy requirements.

To gain:

1 pound of muscle gain

2,500 calories equivalent of 1 pound of muscle,
÷
7 days in a week
=
360 daily excess calories to eat, over maintenance intake number

Note: Intaking calories greater than 1,000 per day **over** the number needed to maintain weight is, however, likely to result in weight gain as body fat, even if you are exercising strenuously on a regular basis.[15]

Caloric Intake Needed To Lose Body Fat

It is physiologically impossible to lose more than two to three pounds of body fat per week.[16] A weight loss greater than this will represent water and lean body tissue. (You'll look lousy, feel weak, be hard to live with, will inherit every germ floating by you, etc., when you drop your **lean** weight.)

To systematically drop that unwanted extra body fat, you need to **drop 3,500 calories a week (or 500 per day) to lose one pound of body fat** and **7,000 calories a week (or 1,000 per day) to lose two pounds of body fat per week.**

To lose:

1 pound fat

3,500 calories
÷
7 days per week
=
500 calories a day less than your maintenance number

To lose:

2 pounds fat

$3,500 \times 2 = 7,000$ calories
÷
7 days per week
=
1,000 calories a day less than your maintenance number

Note: If you desire to drop two pounds a week, but the total caloric intake would be less than 1,200, you need to re-establish your goal and lose only one to one and a half pounds per week. **You never want to eat fewer than 1,200 calories per day.** A daily diet of less than 1,200 calories is likely to be deficient in needed nutrients for you to grow, repair, stay well, and have energy to perform daily tasks and leisure. (Sometimes on a one-to-one basis, a doctor will prescribe a patient to eat fewer than 1,200 calories per day, but he or she will provide extensive guidelines and supplementation. This is **only** under strict supervision of a doctor.)

To lose one or two pounds of fat per week, you need to eliminate 500 or 1,000 calories every day. This reduction can be accomplished by either eating less or exercising more. But remember, for say one hour of aerobics (including the warm-up, aerobic movement, cool-down, and relaxation), you will only use up approximately 300 calories. Is it realistic to think that every day you will engage in two or three **more hours** of endurance exercise (than you now do)? It's highly unlikely for the average individual! Therefore, eliminating 500 or 1,000 calories should predominantly be **eating less food.** If you have yet to develop a fitness program, of course, your elimination of 500 or 1,000 calories per day would come from both the increased exercise (intensity and time duration) **and** eating less food.

Recording Weight Maintenance, Gain, and Loss

Chart 12 has been provided to record your weight maintenance, loss, or gain for a ten-week period.

Summary

If you understand your own basic structure (body type), and makeup (body composition), you can then more accurately set realistic personal appearance goals and goals that lead to your own best cardiorespiratory health.

To maintain a specific weight, your caloric input (eating) must equal your caloric output (daily work and exercise), i.e., it must be **balanced.**

To gain or lose weight, there must be an imbalance of energy. To lose fat, the expenditure has to be a greater number (it takes a loss of 500 cals./day/1 lb. of fat loss); and to facilitate gaining lean, the intake has to be a greater number (it takes adding 360 cals./day/lb. of muscle gain).

To provide a continual means of self-discipline concerning your weight control:

- Assess your weight (Chart 11) whenever any major gain or loss has occurred to your lean or fat;
- Continue setting short and long range goals to achieve or maintain your ideal weight;
- And, monitor your weight for changes (Chart 12), especially if you are prone to having difficulty keeping your weight maintained at your ideal.

Taking time to educate yourself about your own body composition and about how to control your weight can be a very interesting experience. It will provide you with a basis of understanding how the human body physiologically works and how it **doesn't** work.! You can then be alert to all of the false notions, especially of weight loss, that are rampant today. You can develop a program that will work for **you** for a lifetime. And, when it comes to weight control management, consider the following bit of philosophy:

"A person is more motivated to carry out a decision that he has participated in making, than he is a decision that has been imposed upon him by another."[17]

—*Dr. Thomas Gordon*

10

A PROPER DIET TO COMPLETE YOUR TOTAL FITNESS LOOK

"Choose what is best; habit will soon render it agreeable and easy."
—Pythasoras

Nutrients For "Going" and "Growing"

Your body has two basic types of nutrient needs:

- Foods that keep you "going"—the energy needs.
- Foods that keep you "growing"—the growth, repair, and regulation-of-body-processes needs.

Nutrients are chemical substances that your body gets from food during digestion. About fifty nutrients are known to be needed by your body through your diet—"diet" here meaning total intake of food and drink. Essential nutrients are those that your body cannot make or is unable to make in adequate amounts. Therefore, they must be obtained from what you eat and drink. If they are not properly provided for in your diet, your body cannot perform well, mentally or physically.

It Is Your Choice

Just as the opening quotation implies—**choose** what

is best and **habit** will follow—choice is a self-discipline that you must establish. You might know what is "good-for-you" food and "junk" food, but if you don't then **eat** the best choice available, you really don't know good nutrition at all! Good health, optimum fitness, or good nutrition is not just knowing what is right, but doing it.

Good Choice
- A food or drink that provides the nutrients you need to go and grow.

"Junk" Food
- A food that is high in salt, fat, or sugar.

Nutrients Work Together In Teams

The nutrient substances that your body needs can be grouped into the following six categories:

- Proteins.
- Carbohydrates.

- Fats.
- Vitamins.
- Minerals.
- Water.

When you provide all of these categories, each in the proper amounts (called "balancing your diet"), your body will perform like a finely tuned car or precision musical instrument. The movements and sounds could not be sweeter. However, when you decide to establish your own (usually misinformed) needs and priorities and overconsume some nutrients while underconsuming others, you are interfering with the body's balance.

If you know little about human physiology (how the body works), don't resort to just any source for what to eat and how to eat well. There is an abundant quantity of excellent, easy-to-read, scientific literature that has been researched with controls and that will explain what balance of the above nutrients is needed. Read and follow information from established professionals rather than from movie stars or magazines on the supermarket racks. These people are interested in your money. Period.

Supplying the Needs

A well-balanced diet is one that contains the proper amounts of the six basic nutrients, established according to your age, sex, activity level, and state of wellness. Note the following:

- All persons need the same nutrients all their lives but in varying amounts.
- Larger amounts are needed for growth than for maintaining the body.
- Pre-adolescent children need smaller amounts of (food and) nutrients than adults, although they need the same ones.
- Boys and men need and use more nutrients and energy than girls and women.
- The only exception to the above is the need for iron. Women of child-bearing age need more iron than other people.
- Active people require more nutrients that provide energy than inactive people.
- People recovering from illness need more nutrients than when in good health.[1]

These nutrients can be supplied by eating from the four food groups, as illustrated in the pamphlet "Guide to Good Eating, A Recommended Daily Pattern," published by the National Dairy Council.[2] It is not always possible to intake all essential nutrients every twenty-

four hours. What **is** important is that over a span of several days and weeks there is a continual selection from the four groups to meet nutrient needs.

Milk Group

This is the only group that changes (according to the servings you need) in reference to your age. Adults need two servings (except pregnant or lactating women, who need four servings); growing, pre-adolescent children need three servings; and teenagers need four servings. The nutrients involved are needed to build the basic structure and strength of bones and teeth, assist in the production of energy needs, and help in the growth and maintenance of every living cell.

One serving is equal to any of the following choices you make:

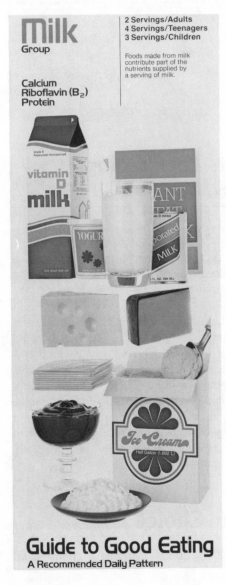

Figure 10-1.

Guide to Good Eating
A Recommended Daily Pattern

1 cup milk (low-fat milk has half the calories)
1 cup yogurt (yogurt is fermented milk)
1 cup pudding
1½ slices (1½ oz.) cheddar cheese ★
1¾ cup (2 big scoops) ice cream (it's not junk food!)
2 cups cottage cheese ★(low-fat=fewer calories of energy intake)

★Count the cheddar cheese and cottage cheese as a serving of milk **or** meat group, but not both simultaneously.[3]

Remember—if you are not an avid "milk" fan, you can eat any of the food in the group and it will supply the calcium, riboflavin, and protein that you need.

Meat Group

This group is called the "meat group," but there are also plant foods that, when eaten together, supply the needed protein, niacin, iron, and thiamin and are then considered an alternative choice to eating meat.

Some of the plant foods that can be combined so that their proteins complement each other (i.e., allow the amino acids to combine to form balanced protein) are: dried beans and whole wheat, dried beans and corn or rice, or peanuts and wheat.[4]

Make your own delicious mix of the following ingredients. It has a crunchy, slightly sweet, slightly salty taste. Purchase each item in one-pound lots (total cost is approximately twelve dollars), mix in a sixteen-quart container, and reseal the mixture in airtight bags. Eating about one-half cup (snack) to one cup (a serving) a day provides an excellent-tasting protein alternative that will last about six weeks. The cost immediately seems reasonable when you price even one steak! And as a snack, it's much more nutritious and cheaper than the costly candy bars and fatty/salty snacks in bags.

Maz Mix

No salt or oil in process:
● Wheat nuts
● Sunflower seeds
● Almonds
● Pecans
● Walnuts (quartered)

Salted and oil in process:
● Dried soybeans
● Sesame sticks

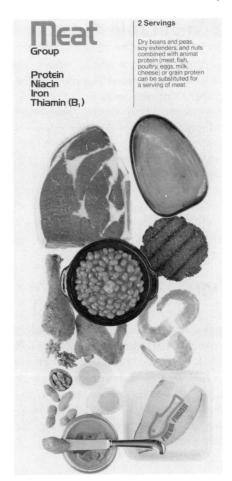

Meat Group

Protein
Niacin
Iron
Thiamin (B₁)

2 Servings

Dry beans and peas, soy extenders, and nuts combined with animal protein (meat, fish, poultry, eggs, milk, cheese) or grain protein can be substituted for a serving of meat.

Figure 10-2.

Box each of:
● Chopped dates coated with oat flour
● Raisins

All persons need two servings per day of the meat group (except pregnant women, who need three servings per day). One serving is equal to: two ounces of cooked lean meat, fish, or poultry. **Or** the protein equivalent would be:

2 eggs
2 slices (2 oz.) cheddar cheese
1 cup dried beans; peas
½ cup cottage cheese
4 Tbs. peanut butter

Note: Count cheeses as servings of meat or milk, but not both simultaneously.[5]

Remember—strip all excess fat off any meat that you eat. Remove the skin from poultry, and eat only the meat. You will thus eliminate unnecessary calories.

Fruit and Vegetable Group

This group provides vitamins A and C, which are actually catalysts or **action starters**. The most important functions of these vitamins include:

- Formation and maintenance of skin and body linings.
- Cementing substances to promote strength in cells and hasten healing of injuries.
- Functions in all visual processes.
- Aids in the use of iron.

These are all functions that you want to enjoy, so be sure not to slight this group.

Sources of Vitamin A

Orange and green. Remembering two simple colors will help you remember that foods of those colors will provide vitamin A. It is recommended that dark green, leafy, or orange vegetables and fruits be eaten at least every other day. Because vitamin A is stored in the fat tissue of the body, an overdose through supplementation in pill form can be fatal. (The same is true for the other fat-soluble vitamins: D, E, and K.)

Sources of Vitamin C

Citrus fruits are recommended daily for supplying the needed catalyst, vitamin C. This vitamin is water-soluble, which means that if too much is intaken, the extra is excreted through the urine, etc. If you decide to take vitamin C supplement pills through massive doses, your body reacts by increasing the level it needs! If you then suddenly stop taking vitamin C supplements, your body reacts as if it were deficient! So supplementation is costly and unnecessary for well persons who eat right.

Servings and Sources of the Fruit and Vegetable Group

All persons need four servings per day. One serving is:

½ cup cooked
½ cup juice
1 cup raw
Medium size apple, banana, etc.[6]

Important sources of this group:

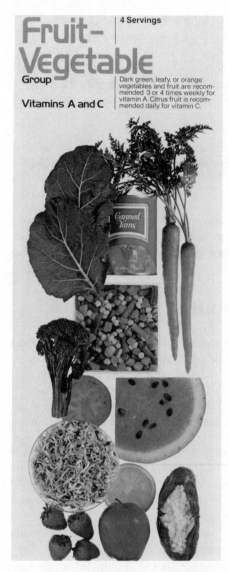

Fruit-Vegetable Group

Vitamins A and C

4 Servings

Dark green, leafy, or orange vegetables and fruit are recommended 3 or 4 times weekly for vitamin A. Citrus fruit is recommended daily for vitamin C.

Figure 10-3.

Vitamin A: carrots, sweet potatoes, greens.
Vitamin C: broccoli, orange, grapefruit, strawberries.

Grain Group (Whole, Fortified, Enriched)

Although this group assists with the growth and maintenance of cells and with the elimination process (fiber provides bulk to your waste for easy removal), the major function is to provide energy! Your number one daily need is energy, to allow you to perform every single daily function, from sleeping to aerobics.

Four servings per day is the minimum amount required by all groups. Remember—if you do not:

- Use this carbohydrate food for the expenditure of energy

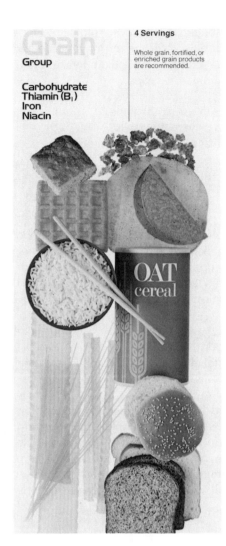

Grain

Group

Carbohydrate
Thiamin (B₁)
Iron
Niacin

4 Servings

Whole grain, fortified, or
enriched grain products
are recommended.

OAT cereal

Figure 10-4.

- Use it for growth and repair or
- Eliminate it,

You **wear it as body fat**—future energy. It's like constantly carrying around extra gasoline for your car.

One serving is equal to:

1 slice bread
½ bun
1 cup cold cereal
½ cup spaghetti or cooked cereal[7]
5 crackers
3 cups popped corn (minus salt and butter)

A minimum amount of four servings was suggested as a daily intake. Look again to see exactly how much a serving is. It is, again, not all you consume or serve yourself at one time, but a **measured amount** of food. If you wish to lose fat weight, watch the amount of additional energy food that you intake. If, however, you are a quite active person—a varsity or endurance athlete—you will **want** to provide an abundance of this energy food four hours before your sport activity.

Special Dietary Guidelines For Americans

Food alone cannot make you healthy. But good eating habits based on moderation and variety can help keep you healthy and even improve your health. The following guidelines suggested for most Americans were developed by the U.S. Department of Agriculture, U.S. Department of Health and Human Services, and printed in more complete detail in the pamphlet, "Nutrition and Your Health."[8] In brief, it is suggested that Americans need to pay more attention to the following:

1
Eat a variety of foods. No single food item supplies all the essential nutrients in the amounts you need. The greater the variety, the less likely you are to develop either a deficiency or an excess of any single nutrient.

2
Maintain ideal weight. If you are too fat, your chances of developing some chronic disorders are increased (i.e., high blood pressure, diabetes, heart attacks, strokes). To lose weight, increase physical activity, eat less fat and fatty foods, eat less sugar and sweets, and avoid too much alcohol.

3
Avoid too much fat, saturated fat, and cholesterol. If you have a high blood cholesterol level, you have a greater chance of having a heart attack. Populations like ours with diets high in saturated fats and cholesterol tend to have high blood cholesterol levels.

There is controversy about what recommendations are appropriate for healthy Americans. But for the U.S. population as a whole, a reduction in our current intake of total fat, saturated fat, and cholesterol is sensible.

To avoid too much fat, saturated fat, and cholesterol:

- Choose lean meats, fish, poultry, dry beans, and peas as your protein sources.
- Moderate your use of eggs and organ meats (such as liver).
- Limit your intake of butter, cream, hydrogenated margarines, shortenings, and coconut oil, and foods made from such products.
- Trim excess fat off meats.

- Broil, bake, or boil rather than fry.
- Read labels carefully to determine both amount and types of fat contained in foods.

4

Eat foods with adequate starch and fiber. The major sources of energy in the average U.S. diet are carbohydrates and fats. Carbohydrates have an advantage over fats: they contain less than half the number of calories per ounce than fats.

Complex carbohydrate foods are better than simple carbohydrates. Simple carbohydrates (sugars) provide calories (for energy) but little else in the way of nutrients. Complex carbohydrates (beans, nuts, fruits, whole grain breads) contain many essential nutrients plus calories for energy.

Increasing your consumption of certain complex carbohydrates can also help increase dietary fiber, which tends to reduce the symptoms of chronic constipation, diverticulosis, and some types of "irritable bowel." There is also concern that diets low in fiber content might also increase the risk of developing cancer of the colon. Eating fruits, vegetables, and whole grain breads and cereals will allow adedquate fiber in the diet.

5

Avoid too much sugar. The major hazard from eating too much sugar is tooth decay. The risk increases:

- With the more frequently you eat sugar and sweets, especially between meals.
- If you eat foods that stick to the teeth (sticky candy, dates, daylong use of soft drinks).

Americans use 130 pounds of sugars and sweeteners a year, each! (Line up twenty-six five-pound empty sugar bags to get the visual effect!)

To avoid excess sugar:

- Use less of all sugars (white, brown, raw, honey, and syrups).
- Select fresh fruit or fruit canned without heavy syrup.
- Read food labels for sugar included—sucrose, glucose, maltose, dextrose, lactose, fructose, or syrup. If it's one of the first ingredients, a lot of sugar is inside.

6

Avoid too much sodium. The major hazard of excessive sodium is how it affects your blood pressure. In populations where high-sodium intake is common, high blood pressure is likewise common. In populations where low-sodium intake occurs, high blood pressure is rare.

High blood pressure is a "forever" problem. Once you have it, you have it for the rest of your life and must **always** then monitor your sodium intake! Establish preventative measures early:

- Eliminate all salt use at the table.
- Cook with no or very little salt.
- Select foods that are low in sodium content.

7

If you drink alcohol, do so in moderation. Alcoholic beverages tend to be high in calories and low in other nutrients. Heavy drinkers may lose their appetites for foods that contain essential nutrients. Vitamin and mineral deficiencies occur commonly in heavy drinkers:

- Because of poor intake.
- Because alcohol alters absorption and use of some essential nutrients.

It has been said that education leads to **moderation** in all areas of life. One or two drinks daily appear to cause no harm in adults. However, even moderate drinkers need to remember that alcohol is a high-calorie, low-nutrient food, and if you wish to achieve or maintain ideal weight, the intake must be monitored.

Nutrition and the Athlete

Guidelines:

The proper food intake of the athlete is the starting point for training or conditioning. The food groups already presented form the **foundation** of the diet recommended for young athletes. This plan serves as the nucleus for meals both in and out of athletic seasons. There is a vast leeway in the choice of the foods within each of the food groups. Major deviations for athletes from these food groups should rarely be necessary. **Basic nutritional needs of athletes and nonathletes do not differ except for caloric needs.**[9]

Total caloric needs vary with individual metabolism and physical activity. An intake of **2000 calories each day should be the bare minimum** allowed for an athlete involved in a vigorous training program. The amount of calories expended by a young male athlete in serious training may range as high as 4000-6000 calories per day. Remember, however, that calorie intake that exceeds expenditure for basal body functions, for physical activity, and for growth of lean body mass, will form body fat!

The Pre-Game Diet:

A pre-game meal should:

- Support blood sugar levels to avoid hunger sensations.
- Leave the stomach and upper bowel empty at the time of competition.
- Provide maximum hydration.
- Minimize stomach upset; promote maximum performance.
- Provide a psychological edge by including foods the athlete likes and believes will make him/her win.

Figure 10-5. Nutrition and the Athlete—Cheerleading, with a 100-pound, one-arm extension press.

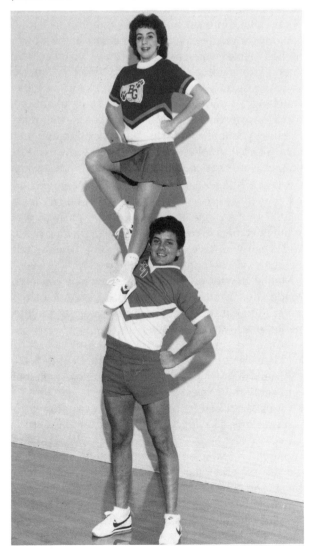

1

Carbohydrates in the diet will support blood sugar and provide glycogen stores to maintain these levels. Glycogen is the storage form of carbohydrate and seems to be the quickest and most efficient source of energy.

Good choices of high carbohydrate foods are: apples, applesauce, bagels, baked potatoes, baking powder biscuits, bananas, boiled potatoes, bread (white, whole wheat), cheese pizza, egg noodles, graham crackers, a hard roll, macaroni and cheese, mashed potatoes, oatmeal, an orange, orange juice, orange sherbet, pancakes (enriched), a pear, spaghetti (cooked), sponge cake, sweet potatoes, and waffles.

2

You may wonder which foods are easily digested and will leave the stomach empty for the competition. Again, **carbohydrates** are more rapidly digested than protein and fat. (A breakfast of toast and jam, cereal with low-fat milk, and fruit or juice will leave the stomach much sooner than a meal of eggs with steak, sausage, or bacon.)

3

Optimum hydration is very important to the athlete, especially to those involved in endurance events, such as long-distance swimming or running. The immediate pre-game diet should consist of **2 to 3 glasses of some beverage**, with no less than eight full glasses each 24 hours.

Whole milk is not recommended because of its high fat content; caffeine should also be avoided because it may increase nervous tension and agitation before the contest. **Non-carbonated fruit drinks** are generally a good choice.

4

Very concentrated sources of simple sugar, such as glucose tablets or undiluted honey, should be avoided, as they can cause gas distention and discomfort. Also, very bulky foods high in fiber or cellulose would not be a good choice before an event.

Heavily salted foods should probably be avoided on the day of competition because they can cause water retention, which decreases athletic performance.

5

The pre-game meal should be eaten from three to four hours before the contest. Here are two sample meals. The first contains approximately 1000 calories and would be ideal for a sport demanding a great deal of energy. The second contains approximately 500 calories and would be ideal for sports demanding lower energy. (Note: One researcher shows that over 70 percent of American Blacks are lactase deficient, which means that they do not have the enzyme to digest milk; you will want to substitute if this affects you.)

Sample Pre-Game Meals[10]

1000 Calories

Milk, skim	2 cups
Hamburger	4 oz. patty
Potatoes, mashed	1 cup
Bread	2 slices, 1 bun
Green beans	½ cup
Fat spread	1 tsp.
Orange (or other fruit)	½ cup or 1 whole
Plain cookies	2

500 calories

Milk, skim	1 cup
Chicken	2 oz.
Potatoes, mashed	1 cup
Bread	2 slices
Fat spread	1 tsp.
Orange (or other fruit)	½ cup or 1 whole

In conclusion, athletes make special demands on their bodies and must be physically prepared to meet those demands.[11] The starting block is sound nutrition knowledge and practice. Don't sacrifice a winning excellence with an inefficient or harmful diet. Reduced strength and endurance, and a poor performance would be your result.

The Psychology of Eating

You eat to fulfill one of two purposes:

- Your hunger (physical need).
- Your appetite (mental need).

To establish a balance in your relationship with food, you must clearly understand **why** you eat **when you do.** To get in touch with this understanding is to truly "know thyself," and, for many people, to then be able to make needed and wanted changes in their overweight or obese bodies.

It was discovered that during a three-year study, nine out of ten persons who took an aerobic dance course were overweight or obese and hoped to lose weight. They felt that with aerobic dancing they would

accomplish this. But the results of monitoring weight changes over an eight-to-ten-week period revealed that only **very few dedicated** persons experienced any significant weight loss during an aerobic dance course.[12] By admission, they simply had not yet made the change in intake patterns both by volume of what was eaten and by selection of what was lower in calories. And they found, as you soon will, that it is easier to eat less food to drop fat weight than it is to exercise it off, although a combination of both **must** be present to establish the proper kind of loss.

Hunger Versus Appetite

Physiologically, when you are hungry, your body will give you cues to "feed me," such as stomach pangs, perhaps a headache, maybe a weak feeling. It's time—time to take a break from the exertion in which you are engaged (work or play), relax, and choose wisely from the varieties of food that you haven't eaten yet today.

Appetite is mental hunger. You smell french fries cooking somewhere; you smell popcorn at the movies or ball game; you pass by a candy machine and "need" some energy; it's noon and you get an "attack" as you pass by a local fast-food restaurant; or you're watching TV and see your favorite food advertised. All of these external cues are mental cues—your mind is telling you that you are in need of food, rather than your internal, or physical cues, which show that true hunger is present and that nourishment is necessary.

Physical hunger can be satisfied by educating yourself toward your body's cues: "Boy, I'm hungry for a salad," or, "A piece of meat for dinner must be part of my next meal!" You seem to crave a specific need. And when you have eaten enough, you have a "full feeling" and can continue with your day.

Mental hunger or appetite can **never** be satisfied. Ponder that a moment. There is no bottom of the barrel. You eat, not listening to physical cues but to mental ones—and they never stop coming.

- "Here's a candy bar. It will make me feel better."
- "I need another glass of pop (coffee, etc.—caffeine) to settle my nerves."
- "I just exercised for a half hour, so I'm going to go reward myself with a big hot fudge sundae!"

Eating and drinking are used to relieve the stress that you are experiencing in life, today. Everyone does this at one time or another, but it is the vast majority of people who **regularly** eat to excess—three times a day plus constant snacking—who have the overweight and obese problem. If you don't want your reaction to stress to show on you like a flag waving help, you must select another outlet for life's daily situations of stress than eating and drinking! Hopefully, you will select a positive outlet like aerobics and relaxation, rather than an equally negative outlet to overeating (smoking, excessive drinking, wife-husband-child abuse, etc.).

Did You Know That . . .

1
Intake of inadequate protein, calcium, and vitamin D in one's quest for slimness, together with low estrogen levels resulting from **excessive,** intense exercise, can produce bone thinning in women and may cause an excessive rate of injury.[13]

2
Plant-derived foods are **always** cholesterol-free.[14]

3
Fish oil not only helps the health of arteries but it also appears to act against inflammation. (It may thus prove useful in many diseases such as arthritis, which is inflammation out of control.)[15]

4
The high fat content of ice cream essentially "protects" the diabetic from rapidly absorbing the sugar.[16]

5
Calcium supplements for post-menopausal women have come to be widely recommended as a way to protect against bone thinning. However, one can't assume that just because a pill is **swallowed,** the calcium in it will be **absorbed** by the intestine. Calcium carbonate is the most widely used preparation and requires the presence of stomach acid for adequate absorption. (An acid-free stomach allows only a small amount of the calcium in the calcium carbonate pill to be absorbed.) The absorption of the calcium is satisfactory if the pill is taken **with a meal**.[17]

Caloric Values of Foods and Beverages

To assist you with your food intake monitoring program on Charts 13 and 14, Tables 10-1 and 10-2 are provided. For your convenience, the individual foods and beverages are listed according to the food group to which they belong.

Table 10-1[18]

Milk Group	Calories	Milk Group (continued)	Calories
Buttermilk, 1 cup	88	Yogurt, Fruit, 1 cup	225
Cheese, American, 1 oz.	104		
Cheese, Cheddar, 1 oz.	113	**Meat and Other Protein-Rich Food Group**	
Cheese, Cottage, ½ cup	120	Bacon, ½ oz.	92
Cheese, Swiss, 1 oz.	103	Beans, Refried, ½ cup	142
Cream, Sour, 1 tbsp.	25	Beef, Roast, 3 oz.	182
Cream, Whipped, 1 tbsp.	26	Beef Liver, 3 oz.	195
Half-and-Half, 1 tbsp.	20	Bologna, 1 oz.	86
Ice Cream, Vanilla, ½ cup	138	Chicken, Fried, 3 oz.	201
Milk, 1 cup	150	Egg, Fried, large	108
Milk, Chocolate, 1 cup	213	Hard-cooked, large	82
Milk, Lowfat (2%), 1 cup	118	Scrambled, large	111
Milk, Skim, 1 cup	77	Frankfurter, 2 oz.	172
Milkshake, Chocolate, 1½ cups	391	Ham, Baked, 3 oz.	179

Meat/Protein Group *(continued)*

	Calories
Meat Loaf, 3 oz.	230
Meat Patty, 3 oz.	186
Peanut Butter, 2 tbsp.	186
Peanuts, Salted, ¼ cup	211
Perch, Fried, Breaded, 3 oz.	193
Pork Chop, 3 oz.	308
Sausage, 1 oz.	135
T-Bone Steak, 3 1/3 oz.	212
Tuna, 3 oz.	168

Fruit-Vegetable Group

Apple, medium	80
Applesauce, ½ cup	116
Apricots, Dried, 4 halves	39
Asparagus, 4 spears, ½ cup	12
Banana, medium	101
Beans, Green, ½ cup	16
Beans, Lima, ½ cup	94
Beets, ½ cup	31
Broccoli, stalk, ½ cup	20
Cabbage, 1/6 head, 1/2 cup	13
Cantaloupe, ¼ medium	29
Carrots, ½ cup	22
Carrot Sticks, 5" carrot	21
Cauliflower, ½ cup	13
Celery Sticks, 8" stalk	10
Coleslaw, ½ cup	82
Corn, ½ cup	70
Corn, 5" ear	114
Fruit Salad, ½ cup, apple, orange, banana, lettuce	99
Grapefruit, pink, ½ medium	48
Grapes, ½ cup	48
Greens, ½ cup, mustard greens, spinach greens, turnip greens	17
Lettuce, 1/6 head, 1/2 cup	10
Lettuce Leaves, 2 large	9
Onions, ½ cup	30
Orange, medium	65
Orange Juice, ½ cup	56
Peaches, ½ cup	100
Pear, medium	101
Peas, Green, ½ cup	54
Pineapple, large slice	90

Fruit-Vegetable Group *(continued)*

	Calories
Potato, Baked, large	132
Potatoes, French-Fried, 20 pieces	233
Potatoes, Mashed, ½ cup	63
Potato, Sweet, ½ medium	78
Raisins, 4½ tbsp.	123
Squash, Summer, ½ cup	16
Squash, Winter, ½ medium, ½ cup	56
Strawberries, ½ cup	28
Tomato, ½ medium	22
Tomato Juice, ½ cup	26
Tossed Salad, ¾ cup, lettuce, green pepper, radish, carrot	13
Watermelon, 1 cup	52

Grain Group

Bagel	165
Biscuit	103
Bread, White, slice	61
Bread, Whole Wheat, slice	55
Cornbread, 2½" x 3"	191
Corn Flakes, ¾ cup	72
Crackers, Graham, 2	54
Crackers, Saltines, 5	60
Noodles, Egg, ½ cup	100
Oatmeal, ½ cup	66
Pancake, 4"	61
Popcorn, plain, 3 cups	69
Rice, ½ cup	112
Roll, Frankfurter/Hamburger	119
Tortilla, Corn, 6"	63
Waffles, 2, 3½" x 5½"	130

Others

Bar, Milk Chocolate, 1 oz.	147
Beer, 1½ cups, 12 oz.	151
Butter, 1 tsp.	36
Cake, Devil's Food, 1/16 of 9" cake	234
Chocolate Syrup, 2 tbsp.	93
Cookie, Sugar, 3" diameter	89
Highball, 1½ oz. whiskey, gin, rum, or vodka, with soda	97
Mayonnaise, 1 tbsp.	101
Pie, Apple, 1/6 of 9" pie	403
Roll, Danish Pastry	274
Sugar, 1 tsp.	14
Wine, Rosé, 3½ oz.	87

Table 10-2[19]

Caloric Values of Fast Foods

BURGER CHEF	Calories
Big Shef	542
Cheeseburger	304
Double Cheeseburger	434
French Fries	187
Hamburger, Regular	258
Mariner Platter	680
Rancher Platter	640
Shake	326
Skipper's Treat	604
Super Shef	600

BURGER KING	
Cheeseburger	305
Hamburger	252
Whopper	606
French Fries	214
Vanilla Shake	332
Whaler	486
Hot Dog	291

McDONALD'S	
Egg McMuffin	352
English Muffin, Buttered	186
Hot Cakes, W/Butter & Syrup	472
Sausage (Pork)	184
Scrambled Eggs	162
Big Mac	541
Cheeseburger	306
Filet O Fish	402
French Fries	211
Hamburger	257
Quarter Pounder	418
Quarter Pounder W/Cheese	518
Apple Pie	300
Cherry Pie	298
McDonaldland Cookies	294
Chocolate Shake	364
Strawberry Shake	345
Vanilla Shake	323

DAIRY QUEEN	
Big Brazier Deluxe	470
Big Brazier Regular	457
Big Brazier W/Cheese	553
Brazier W/Cheese	318
Brazier Cheese Dog	330
Brazier Chili Dog	330
Brazier Dog	273
Brazier French Fries, 2.5 oz.	200
Brazier French Fries, 4.0 oz.	320
Brazier Onion Rings	300
Brazier Regular	260
Fish Sandwich	400

DAIRY QUEEN (cont.)	Calories
Fish Sandwich w/Cheese	440
Super Brazier	783
Super Brazier Dog	518
Super Brazier Dog W/Cheese	593
Super Brazier Chili Dog	555
Banana Split	540
Buster Bar	390
DQ Chocolate Dipped Cone, med	300
DQ Chocolate Dipped Cone, lg	450
DQ Chocolate Malt, sm	340
DQ Chocolate Malt, med	600
DQ Chocolate Malt, lg	840
DQ Chocolate Sundae, sm	170
DQ Chocolate Sundae, med	300
DQ Chocolate Sundae, lg	400
DQ Cone, sm	110
DQ Cone, med	230
DQ Cone, lg	340
Dairy Queen Parfait	460
Dilly Bar	240
DQ Float	330
DQ Freeze	520
DQ Sandwich	140
Fiesta Sundae	570
Hot Fudge Brownie Delight	570
Mr. Misty Float	440
Mr. Misty Freeze	500

KENTUCKY FRIED CHICKEN	
Original Recipe Dinner*	830
Extra Crispy Dinner*	950
Individual Pieces† (Original Recipe)	
Drumstick	136
Keel	283
Rib	241
Thigh	276
Wing	151
9 Pieces	1892

LONG JOHN SILVER'S	
Breaded Oysters, 6 pc.	460
Breaded Clams, 5 oz.	465
Chicken Planks, 4 pc.	458
Cole Slaw, 4 oz.	138
Corn on Cob, 1 pc.	174
Fish W/Batter, 2 pc.	318

LONG JOHN SILVER'S (cont.)	
Fish W/Batter, 3 pc.	477
Fryes, 3 oz.	275
Hush Puppies, 3 pc.	153
Ocean Scallops, 6 pc.	257
Peg Leg W/Batter, 5 pc.	514
Shrimp W/Batter, 6 pc.	269
Treasure Chest 2 pc. fish, 2 Peg Legs	467

PIZZA HUT**	
Thin 'N Crispy	
Beef†	490
Pork†	520
Cheese	450
Pepperoni	430
Supreme	510
Thick 'N Chewy	
Beef†	620
Pork†	640
Cheese	560
Pepperoni	560
Supreme	640

TACO BELL	
Bean Burrito	343
Beef Burrito	466
Beefy Tostada	291
Bellbeefer	221
Bellbeefer W/Cheese	278
Burrito Supreme	457
Combination Burrito	404
Enchirito	454
Pintos 'N Cheese	168
Taco	186
Tostada	179

BEVERAGES	
Coffee, 6 oz.	2
Tea, 6 oz.	2
Orange Juice, 6 oz.	56
Chocolate Milk, 8 oz.	213
Skim Milk, 8 oz.	77
Whole Milk, 8 oz.	150
Coca-Cola, 8 oz.	96
Fanta Ginger Ale, 8 oz.	84
Fanta Grape, 8 oz.	114
Fanta Orange, 8 oz.	117
Fanta Root Beer, 8 oz.	103
Mr. Pibb, 8 oz.	93
Mr. Pibb without Sugar, 8 oz.	1
Sprite, 8 oz.	95
Sprite without Sugar, 8 oz.	3
Tab, 8 oz.	tr
Fresca, 8 oz.	2

NOTE: Dairy Queen stores in the State of Texas do not conform to Dairy Queen-approved products. Any nutritional information shown does not necessarily pertain to their products.

*Dinner comprises mashed potatoes and gravy, cole slaw, roll, and three pieces of chicken, either 1) wing, rib, and thigh; 2) wing, drumstick, and thigh; or 3) wing, drumstick, and keel.

**Based on a serving size of one half of a 10-inch pizza (3 slices).

†Topping mixture of ingredients.

11

SPECIAL CONCERNS AND MISCONCEPTIONS

As you go through life, you very likely, at one point or another, may find the need to reclassify yourself from a "regular population of aerobic dancers" category with virtually no limitations, to one who now possesses a special need, or concern. This chapter is dedicated to all of those fantastic individuals who are physically overcoming the **limitations** barrier because of less-than-an-optimum bodily condition.

Special Concerns

Your body functions in predictable ways over 90 percent of the time. If you understand cause, effect, and therefore **prevention**, you are going to find that exercising your body is not a drudgery of pain and injuries, but a joy—a release, an outlet, a diversion for the mental and emotional stress in your life. It feels good to be so "tuned in" to your own physiological needs that your risk of injury is low. This "tuning in" is not a mystical phenomenon, but comes about by **educating** yourself about how the body works and how it doesn't work.

If you have systematically developed your aerobic dance program as outlined in this text, chapter by chapter, you will have discovered an excellent way in which to develop your total fitness. If the assessments, guidelines, and techniques were carefully followed, your chance for problems and injuries will have been greatly reduced!

Care and Prevention of Program-Related Injuries

The following are the more common program-related problems that you may incur. Again, understanding prevention before the occurrence is the key to a safe and comfortable program hour.

Apparel and Injury

1

As previously detailed, proper shoes are your number one concern. When you jump or run, you place three to six times more force on your feet than when you are stationary. If you weigh 125 pounds, this means that you are placing 375 to 750 pounds of pressure on your feet with each jump or run. Your body can withstand the stress of exercise better if this extra pressure is "shock absorbed" by the shoe you wear, or the giving quality of the surface upon which you move. Select a shoe that totally supports your foot for aerobic dance. Criteria are listed in Chapter 2. Dance preferably on wood to all other surfaces. "Ideal floor surface is hardwood suspended on springs over an air space."[1]

And when it's time to get a new pair of shoes, do it! The inside of the shoe deteriorates first, so gauge your buying by when the inside wears out, not by how the rubber on the sole, etc. wears.

2

You want to prevent friction, so wear cotton socks that absorb sweat and have no wrinkles.

3

"Leg warmers" (heavy, very bulky long socks that you will see performance dancers wear in-between performances) are for just that purpose. During the warm-up phase of the aerobic dance hour, you may wish to wear these in cooler weather. However, while you are dancing, or in warm weather, do not wear them. You want to be able to sweat and allow your cooling mechanism to function properly. In order to sweat freely, you must allow the sweat to be on your skin, exposed to the air. Leg warmers will absorb sweat and not allow the cooling mechanism to function properly. When you superficially heat the skin for a duration of time, it retains the internal body heat and soon causes heat exhaustion or even heat stroke. You do not want to interfere with your body's cooling mechanism by the use of stylish fad apparel of any kind (the same principles apply to the use of sweatshirts and pants).

4

Tights or nylon hosiery are sometimes worn by women to aesthetically make their legs look better by hiding the fat or flaws located there. The only time that either (tights, nylons, etc.) should be worn is in **cold** weather to retain the body heat. Again, nylon materials (of which tights and nylon hosiery are made) retain body heat. In warm weather you must allow the legs to sweat freely by exposing the skin surface directly to **air.** Don't be embarrassed by how your legs look—at least you are **working on improvement** by aerobic dancing!

5

Finally, it is against all physiological principles to wear a towel around the neck during exercise. The major artery from the heart to the brain is located in the neck area and needs to be able to be cooled by exposure of the skin surface in that area to air.

Water Intake

Being **able** to perform aerobic dance depends upon the replacement of your water losses. Water serves as the principle means of transporting heat (and substances) within the body. In warm environments (meaning within a room or a geographical location), it is the **only** means of dispersing body heat. This is accomplished by the evaporation of released perspiration on the surface of the skin. When the room air contacts the sweat, the skin surface is cooled, and the cooling is then internally conducted.

The production of body heat is greatly increased during physical exercise. **Unless water for perspiration is available, the body temperature increases beyond normal and there is overheating.** Thus, when fluid loss exceeds supply, dehydration follows, with an accompanying limited ability to exercise. When dehydration occurs, even modest physical activity causes the **heart rate and body temperature to increase.** When the water loss is approximately 5 percent of the total body water, evidence of heat exhaustion may become apparent, and when losses total 10 percent, the condition may soon lead to heat stroke, which is fatal unless cared for immediately (i.e., an ice bath submersion).

It is imperative that fluid intake be increased to maintain fluid balance as the work level and environmental temperature increase.[2]

Since there is no basis for restricting water intake during an aerobic dance hour and no evidence that humans can "adapt" or be "trained" to tolerate water intake that is lower than your daily losses, you should practice the habit of replacing water loss by continuous daily fluid intake.

Here are a few guidelines to facilitate water balance:

1

Drink plenty of liquids at least twenty minutes before the beginning of an aerobic hour. Frequent small intakes of fluid throughout the day is best.

2

For most sessions, if you have been providing plenty of water **prior** to the aerobic dance hour, you probably will not need to intake water **during** the hour (room temperature and humidity are the variables that usually determine this.) However, if you get thirsty during an hour, **do not hesitate to drink water.** Your thirst mechanism is even a **late** sign that you need water, so don't ignore it!

3

After an aerobic hour, relax and sit with a tall glass of ice water or lemonade. This will provide immediate rehydration and is a pleasant way to conclude your hour "to yourself."

Deliberate dehydration (by loading on the clothes and promoting profuse sweating), of course, is not an acceptable method for weight control. This will cause a temporary loss of weight that is **rapidly regained by rehydration.** Loss of weight should only be body fat, **never** water or protein.

Blisters

Blisters come in seconds and take days to heal. Even a small blister that goes uncared for will bother your workout. The best advice is to do everything you can to prevent them from forming.

Blisters are caused by friction—a surface of your shoe rubbing against the skin of your foot. Make sure that your shoes fit well—not too loose, not too tight. To assist in the prevention of blisters, one simple procedure is to lubricate the trouble spot with petroleum jelly before you put your shoes on for another fitness hour. If you sweat a lot, powder your feet also. Improper-fitting shoes are the culprit, so be sure that you do a few exertive moves in your local shoe store to size up comfort **in motion** before you purchase the shoes.

If you get a water blister, care for it as follows:

1
Gently scrub the area with soap and water to thoroughly clean the area.

2
Gently swab with alcohol or a surgical preparation.

3
Make two incisions at the outer edges of the blister. Slowly press out the superficial fluid. Apply ointment or first-aid cream and bandage until healed completely.

If you get a blood blister, care for it as follows:

1
Ice the area.

2
Do not puncture. The chance of infection is great, since you immediately are in connection with your circulatory system.

3
Place a "donut"-type compress around the blister until it is reabsorbed and completely healed.

Bunions

A bunion is a large bony protuberance on the outside of the big toe that indicates joint inflammation. The principle causes of bunions are overpronation and faulty foot structure. Seeking correction from a podiatrist is your plan of action.

Cramps (Muscle)

A cramp is a painful spasm of muscle. Cramping may occur during or following a vigorous exercise session and is the result of two different phenomena. Muscle cramping **during** an exercise session is primarily due to an electrolyte and fluid imbalance in your system.[3] Electrolytes are sodium, calcium, chloride, potassium, and magnesium. Cramping occurs primarily because you have not, with regularity, properly replaced your water intake as you condition and train.

If a great deal of sweating has occurred (eight or more pounds of water), replacement of those elements may be obtained by drinking, in solution (never in tablet form), a substance that replaces them. With moderate sweating and water loss, regular, daily water intake and proper diet will replace the needed fluids and electrolyte elements and do much to eliminate this type of cramping.

The most common cramps associated with exercise are those that occur in the **twenty-four hours after** exercise, especially after having gone to bed and/or after a sudden movement. These cramps (postexercise) are not associated with electrolyte imbalance.[4] They are believed to be caused by muscle fiber swelling, causing then the agitation of (peripheral) nerves servicing the muscle tissue. If these cramps are frequent and severe, treatment is usually prescribed by taking .2 grams of quinine sulfate.

Immediate relief for either type of cramping is to **static stretch in the exact opposite direction** for a few moments.

Night Leg Cramps

Night leg cramps are usually caused by the position of the foot (bent down). Prescription: stretching exercises during the day and sleep positions which allow the foot to remain perpendicular to the leg.[5]

Side Stitch

A side stitch is the sharp pain in the side and usually represents a spasm of the diaphragm, the lower portion of the breathing mechanism. It is believed that side stitches occur primarily because not enough oxygen is getting to the area. This is due to a decreased blood flow to the location and most frequently occurs in those who have recently had a meal or drunk large volumes of fluid.

To help alleviate this phenomenon, immediately inhale deeply and bend forward from the waist, making the stomach and intestines push up against the diaphragm, using either a sitting (Figure 11-1) or standing position. Then, "tune in" to your breathing and consciously control your exhale. Do this by forming your lips as if you were going to whistle, and exhale through your puckered lips about five to ten times. For some, this seems to help.

The more conditioned person rarely experiences this type of pain, so prevention lies in continuing your

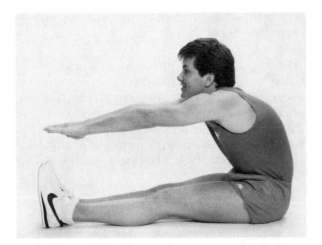

Figure 11-1.

program with regularity, with special attention to strength activities for the abdominal area.

Muscle Soreness

Two types of pain are associated with severe muscular exercise: (1) pain during and immediately after exercise, which may persist for several hours, and (2) a localized soreness that usually does not appear for twenty-four to forty-eight hours. The first is associated with the presence of metabolic wastes on pain receptors, the second with torn muscle fibers and/or connective tissue.[6] The immediate type need not be cause for great concern—it presents no lasting problems. *The delayed type needs* attention in the form of a more adequate warm-up and cool-down stretching program, and the incorporation of concluding strength activities. Gradual, sensible muscle use during exercise is the best prevention.

Muscle, Tendon, and Joint Injuries

1
For **muscle strains or sprains,** you I.C.E.: ICE, COM-

PRESS, AND ELEVATE. Injuries are iced (or cold whirlpools are administered) to inhibit swelling and promote healing by making the body internally (rather than at the surface) supply more blood to the affected deep-problem area. The body forces more blood to come to the area when cold applications are applied by making the body work harder pumping away the old cells and pumping in fresh oxygen and nutrients to begin the repair process at the deep site rather than at the surface skin area. Ice applications are administered two times a day for about twenty minutes. When the affected area no longer is warm to the touch (using the back of your hand), but seems to be the same temperature as the rest of the leg, arm, etc., ice compresses can be stopped.

When heat is applied, it brings an increase of blood to the skin surface, but it doesn't make the body work hard at all—on its own—to pump in a fresh supply of oxygen and nutrients to the **deep** affected area. So stick with the less comfortable ice measure, and your repair process will quicken.

2
Anchilles tendonitis is an inflammation of the thick tendon that connects the heel to the calf muscle. This injury is due to the use of shoes with inadequately thick heels, or which for some other reason do not provide a proper cushion for the foot. Biomechanical problems like the following aggravate the situation: bowed legs, tight hamstrings and calves, high-arched rigid feet, overpronation, and excessive toe-running.

To prevent Achilles tendonitis, perform adequate heel-cord stretching, and **don't exercise** with the pain. Aggravation of this problem can cause a serious and permanent condition.

Shin Splints

The most frequent injury experienced by new aerobics enthusiasts is shin splints. The following information was provided by Jane Steinberg, former athletic trainer for intercollegiate sports at Bowling Green State University, Ohio.

"Shin splints is the term given to pain felt on the **front** and **inside of the lower leg** (Figure 11-2). Although a common affliction of runners, this malady can affect anyone who engages in physical activity which uses the legs. Most cases of shin splints occur in the **beginning** of an exercise program because the lower leg muscles are weak.

Jumping and running activities cause the leg muscles in the back of the leg to develop and become stronger, while the leg muscles in front develop only slightly. This **muscle imbalance** can cause the disabl-

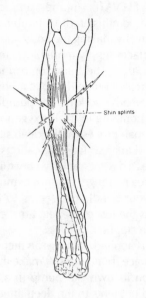

Figure 11-2.

ing pain called 'shin splints' if not treated correctly."[7]

"When the strength of one muscle or muscle group is disproportionate to that of the antagonist(s) for that muscle or group, the weaker muscle should be strengthened to restore balance around the joint."[8]

Preventative measures are the first step with any

exercise regimen. Light, flexible shoes with good arch support are mandatory. Stretching before and after physical activity also helps the muscles absorb shock. Avoid track running; the repeated turns put great stress on the lower leg.

Performing three repetitions of straight-leg and bent-knee wall leans for twenty seconds may help alleviate the problem (Figure 11-3).

Or another preventative measure is to develop the strength of the anterior lower leg area. This can be accomplished by performing an exercise like the lower-leg flexor, which uses two-to-four-pound weights.

Sit, supported by your hands, on a stool or high bench, with your legs hanging down. Place a two-, three-, or four-pound weight over your toes. Sandbags placed over the toes or "Heavy Hands" worn over the toes are two possibilities (Figure 11-4). Flex your feet at the ankle by drawing your toes up tightly toward your knees (Figure 11-5). Return to the starting position

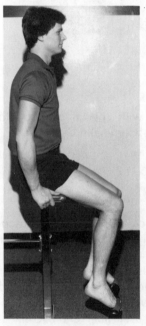
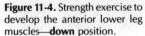
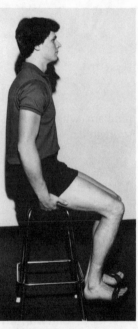

Figure 11-4. Strength exercise to develop the anterior lower leg muscles—**down** position.

Figure 11-5. Strength exercise to develop the anterior lower leg muscles—**up** position.

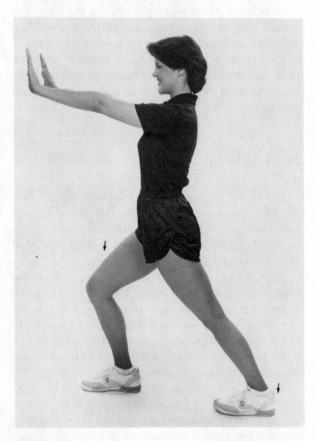

Figure 11-3.

and repeat for one or two minutes by flexing up slowly and lowering toes slowly. This exercise can be done one leg at a time, or both feet working together simultaneously.

Of utmost importance in the caring for shin splints are **rest and immediately icing** the area of tenderness.

The icing should be done for eight to ten continuous minutes by means of gently massaging the problem area. Later in the day, a second gentle ice massage for the same duration of time should begin to give the desired relief. Continue this procedure for several days. You'll be amazed how quickly you "repair" within one week!

Also, you can minimize the discomfort by taking four to six aspirin a day. Toe raises on the edge of a step can help strengthen the posterior muscles which are heavily used in any running, jumping, or dancing activity. Walking on your heels with your toes in the air for thirty to sixty seconds is an easy way to build up strength in the front leg muscles. Pressing down on the heel of the fully extended leg while cycling also helps. Practice this stretch at traffic lights when you must wait.

If icing, rest, aspirin, strengthening, and stretching do not create relief within ten days, see a physician to rule out the more serious conditions such as stress fractures, structural imbalances which might require orthotics, or anterior compartment syndrome.[9]

Structural Imbalances

The **sports orthotics** just mentioned are devices which are custom-made by hand to specifically control the function of your particular foot. (See the photo in Chapter 2.) They are not arch supports. Requiring several weeks of construction, they are shaped to closely **control your foot the entire time it is on the ground.** The bones in your foot are now moved so that muscles can function and adapt normally, decreasing or eliminating foot problems. They are made of an unbreakable, reinforced material and are worn inside of your athletic shoe.[10]

So don't just live with the pain that structural imbalances cause, like aching on the entire bottom of the foot from the forward movement of running, or shin splints from the lateral movement of aerobic dance. You should seek the advice of a qualified specialist like a podiatrist before wearing sports orthotics.

Drug Usage and Potentially Fatal Effects on the Heart

It is believed that as many as half of all heart attack deaths occur because of "electrical failure" of the heart, not "pump failure." People with perfectly adequate amounts of heart muscle die because their heart's electrical signals go out of sync; the muscle then twitches chaotically and can no longer pump blood. Known as **ventricular fibrillation**, this rhythm disturbance is absolutely deadly if it cannot be reversed within minutes.[11] Drug-related deaths of superstar athletes (i.e., cocaine intoxication of recent years) is directly related to this phenomenon.

Female Only Concerns

1

To eliminate breast soreness due to the jogging-type movements performed, wear a **tight** bra (or jogging bra), and cover nipples with soft padding. Full-figured girls and women will find that a good supportive bra will do much to keep the breasts from early sagging, which is caused by the stretching of the connective tissue that provides the breast uplift. If you choose to wear a swimsuit for aerobic dance, again, remember to provide bra support. Complete guidelines in regards to sports bras follow.

As strange as it may sound, an Ace bandage can do a good job of immobilizing breasts. The new bras stop breast movement by flattening breasts rather than shaping them, as conventional bras do. Because of their design and fabrics, some of these new bras can be worn alone. Whether you need to wear a bra at all, and whether you should choose a bra made specifically for aerobic dance depends on your breasts. If aerobic dancing and running makes them sore, or you'd like to stop movement for modesty's sake, a running bra can help. You may only need to wear one before your period or during pregnancy and nursing. And, if you've been running braless without any soreness, you may not want to—or have to—change.

A bra should be comfortable and supportive:

● Straps should let arms swing and shouldn't fall over the shoulders.
● Sides and back of bra should allow the rib cage to expand and contract.
● Cups should prevent breast motion.
● Bra fabric must not be too heavy or bulky, and it must absorb and dissipate sweat.
● If a bra has elastic straps, you'll get lots of bounce.
● Avoid stretch in both straps and cups. Like stretch straps, a stretch cup will give and allow your breasts to move. Horizontal stretch across your body may add comfort, but you should avoid vertical stretch, which will let breasts bounce.
● If the bra doesn't have traditional cups, elasticity plays an even greater role. . . . They rely on the bra's fabric to hold the breasts close, flattening them. The most supportive of these bras have almost no elasticity.
● If you're an A-B- or C-cup and can give up some

support in favor of comfort, look for bras with elasticity in areas that don't directly affect support, i.e., have fully elastic backs. These gain support through non-elastic straps and cups.

Flatter is better. Cups or no cups, look for a bra that reduces your profile. The bra should distribute your breast mass over your chest well rather than shape your breasts to project away from your body. The result of this reduced profile is that there is less mass for gravity to pull against.

- Cups must be wide so your breasts have room to spread over your chest wall.
- Bras that flatten are criticized as unfeminine by women who wear C-cup or smaller bras. As women get larger, they are willing to give up femininity for support.
- The most supportive bras may be tight and constricting, but larger-breasted women have a different perception of tightness because it's the only way they can get enough support.
- Wide straps distribute weight and won't dig into your shoulders. Straps that join toward the center of the back of the bra are less likely to fall down over your shoulders.
- Velcro strips for adjustability is better than clips or hooks.
- Rough-edged seams should be eliminated or kept away from the skin. Sewing the bras inside out to keep seams and hardware away from skin is a helpful manufacturer's technique.

Fabric content:

- Many depend on a heavy nylon/Lycra fabric for support.
- Look for cotton and polypropylene blend and soft cotton lining on the undersides of straps and inside cups.
- Mesh between the cups allows the collection of moisture to evaporate. The racerback bras made of stretch mesh on the back also help.
- Size D-cup or larger—almost entire bra is non-elastic, so it is effective in stopping breast movement.[12]

2

A second female-only concern is this. Vigorous exercise will not make a woman's pelvic organs fall out or be damaged.[13]

3

Concerning that normal, monthly occurrence, the menstrual period—a program of physical exercise will probably help the occasional problem of menstrual cramps.[14] Circulation to the area is greatly increased with vigorous exercise, and therefore congestion is greatly eliminated, assisting in the alleviation of that uncomfortable feeling.

Also, exercises specifically designed for alleviating cramps are of **less** value than simply **practicing good habits of physical fitness and nutrition.**[15]

4

Menstrual abnormality (lighter flow, missed periods) is not unusual in endurance athletes. Some biochemical studies suggest that physical training affects the body's hormones, i.e., ovulation seems to decrease among runners.

Pregnancy

Each woman should check first with her obstetrician/gynecologist and get this doctor's opinion on each individual case. Many doctors prescribe to this rule of exercise: You should be able to continue a program in which you have currently been engaged **before** pregnancy. If you have been involved in aerobic dancing (or jogging, swimming, cycling, etc.), you should be able to continue, but at a noncompetitive, lower intensity (pace of activity) level than previously done. This means less hopping, fewer lower leg and arm movements, and doing more stationary rather than spacial movements.

Dr. Michael Newton, M.D., professor of obstetrics and gynecology at Northwestern Medical School and past director of gynecologic oncology at Prentice Women's Hospital and Maternity Center in Chicago, has enumerated the following guidelines to pregnant women:

1

If you have, prior to pregnancy, been engaged in an aerobic activity you wish to continue, are in good physical condition, and do not engage in competition, there is no reason why you should not continue your exercise program.

2

It is necessary to have an adequate diet, with emphasis on protein, along with some supplementary vitamins and minerals.

3

Physical ability decreases fairly rapidly even before the baby's increasing size makes great exertion impossible, so your intensity level will have to drop markably to coincide with this decreased ability.

4

Nonactive women are advised **against** taking up a new sport or activity during pregnancy, mainly because they would be using unaccustomed muscles and taking a greater chance of getting hurt because they will not have the necessary skills. However, if a woman is already athletically inclined and in good physical condition, there is no reason why she cannot take up a new sport in a moderate, noncompetitive fashion.

5

(Aerobic) swimming is a good exercise for the pregnant woman because so little pressure is exerted on the body, and it can be continued almost until the end of pregnancy.

6

Special problems that women experience during pregnancy are dizziness and the need to empty the bladder frequently. In later months, as the breasts become heavier, good bra support during exercise would become even more important. Increased lower back curvature occurs about the fifth month, with the increasing weight of the baby. Since your center of gravity is shifted forward, activities involving sudden movement might have to be reduced.

7

During the seventh month of pregnancy, the pelvic joints usually tend to become relaxed due to the rising levels of pregnancy hormones, especially progesterone, and some restrictions on activity would then become advisable.

8

Lactating women can continue exercise programs, beginning about three to four weeks after delivery. Women are urged to keep up an adequate fluid intake and a good diet.

9

Women who have Caesarean section can resume aerobic activities within four to six weeks of delivery, provided that their resumption of activity proceeds slowly.[16]

10

"Moderate exercise is well tolerated by the mother and her fetus. Extreme and prolonged exercise, i.e., 40 minutes at 70 percent maximum oxygen consumption, has its greatest risks of **hyperthermia** at 17 to 40 days post-conception and of low birthweight in the third trimester when venous return is limited by weight bearing exercise. Patients at high risk of fetal or maternal compromise should limit exercise."[17]

From these general observations, the following clinical guidelines are useful for the average pregnant woman:

- Consider switching to non-weight-bearing exercise such as swimming, cycling, or rowing, especially in the third trimester.
- Exercise regularly, at least three times a week.
- Limit activity to shorter intervals: exercise ten to fifteen minutes, rest to a pulse rate less than ninety, then exercise for another ten to fifteen minutes.
- Decrease exercise level in the third trimester.
- Monitor the intensity of the exercise. Ideally, exercise should be maintained at 50 to 70 percent maximum oxygen consumption. The target zone concept is useful and can be approximated by measuring heart rate or ventilatory response. Heart rate should be 60 to 80 percent of maximum rate (120 to 140). Ventilatory target zone is approximated by the ability to talk but not to sing comfortably while exercising.[18]

Many physicians are finding tremendous advantages in a good exercise program during pregnancy, since there are increased physiological and emotional demands on the body. A widely accepted aerobics program that is promoted by many physicians is walking. Make it aerobic by walking at the specific heart rate that is within your training zone, and you will have provided yourself with another option!

Several years ago, a study of Olympic women athletes showed that, overall, they had normal pregnancies and that no special risks or dangers were involved. Their improved muscle tone permitted them to complete the second, or expulsion, stage of labor more rapidly than other women. Recovery from childbirth was also better, partly because of the good dietary habits that these women had developed before pregnancy. (Some athletes have performed very well in the early months; however, Olympic-level competition is not practical during pregnancy.)[19]

Also, of late, some researchers have shown that aerobic activity (primarily joggers have been studied) may reduce the menstrual flow or show a marked absence in some females. If you are interested in childbearing, you may wish to consider this finding when beginning an aerobics program.

Seek the Professionals

Understanding the cause and effect will help you to prevent problems or injuries during your quest for fitness. Whenever problems or injuries do occur, don't just "live with it." Seek out answers from the qualified professionals—medical doctors, sports medicine specialists and physiologists, or athletic trainers.

Misconceptions about Fitness

Within any body of information, misconceptions arise from unresearched statements promoted by individuals **not qualified** to make the statements. Many of the myths about the harm that exercise supposedly causes, or unscientific ideas concerning proper diet and exercise programs are being put to rest through better education.

For instance, several persons who are TV and movie personalities talk about "go for the burn." Key fitness research professionals have stated the opposite. "Don't try to achieve what some aerobic programs call the 'burn.' A burning sensation in the chest could mean heart or coronary problems. If other muscles feel as if they were burning, it's probably a signal of overwork or injury approaching!"[20]

This text has been written to assist you, the novice, in understanding how your body works and how to improve it in various unique ways. Its design is purely educational in nature. It will provide you with a firm base so that **you** can evaluate the various programs and products being highly promoted these days in the areas of diet, exercise, and relaxation.

The hope for your ongoing commitment to fitness is that you will refer to the most qualified sources available to answer your continual questions. People who are medical doctors (especially those "wellness" and "preventive medicine" oriented), physiologists and sports medicine specialists, i.e., **the professionals who devote their entire working day and lives to researching and understanding human physiology**—are overwhelmingly more qualified to advise you on a diet, exercise, and relaxation program than a commercially oriented person. Glamorous movie and TV personalities sell you on their "expertise" by their media notoriety, their photogenic bodies and smiles, and the price tag attached to their information.

So be selective. Follow the diet, exercise, and relaxation programs promoted by the **scientific professionals**. Choose to read and believe authors whose credentials are impressive in the various fields of total fitness and who publish their researched findings in **professional journals**. You will then have provided yourself with the most accurate, up-to-date knowledge available, and a more safe, fun way to good health.

12

EVALUATING YOUR AEROBIC DANCE PROGRAM

A Final Thought . . .

Self-discipline is a choice that you make. The key to sticking to a fitness program is to choose flexibility, aerobic, and strength training activities that you truly enjoy and in which you can participate with enthusiasm on a regular basis **for a lifetime. Desire and consistency** are the key words which will provide a firm foundation for your new fitness habits to develop.

It takes hard work to achieve total fitness. There are no shortcuts or easy ways. The less fit you are, the longer it will take to achieve this fitness. You will need to count your progress by months as well as days by means of a continual monitoring program as provided in this text. **Maintaining** fitness, however, is a lot easier than initially **achieving** it. Fitness simply requires self-discipline and choices. Good luck!

Commitment Equals Priority

You **have** time for the priorities in your life. Start right now and establish a plan for prioritizing and incorporating all the phases of total fitness into your current life-style. Having used this text, you should already have a running start on ideas how to do this! What is suggested here is what **follows** your fitness course program . . . steps to insure an ongoing lifetime top-priority commitment.

Begin with a **re-assessment** of all the areas tested earlier to determine how much you've improved or changed from the pre-assessment. **This alone** is usually the most influential incentive for continuing a commitment to fitness for a lifetime.

Next, evaluate your entire program in terms of your **needs/ choices** that must be considered in order for any program phase to be realistically "successful."

And finally, set new attainable **concrete goals** in each fitness area—both short and long term. Without a few set concrete goals to strive toward, a program may lose its spark for enthusiasm! (Half the pleasure in any event in life is the working toward attaining the end result!) "Nothing difficult is ever easy," a wise philosopher once said, but it can be **fun** if there's a challenge to it!

References

Chapter 1

1. Kenneth H. Cooper, M.D., M.P.H., *Running Without Fear*. (New York: M. Evans and Company, Inc., 1985), p. 195.
2. Ibid.
3. American College of Obstetricians and Gynecologists: *Safety Guidelines for Women Who Exercise* (ACOG Home Exercise Programs). Washington, D.C., ACOG, 1986, p.6.
4. Kenneth H. Cooper, Movie, "Run Dick, Run Jane," Brigham Young University, Provo, Utah, 1971.
5. Cooper, *Running Without Fear*, p. 128.
6. Ibid., p. 192.
7. Ibid., p. 197.
8. Kenneth H. Cooper, M.D., M.P.H. *The Aerobics Program for Total Well-Being*. (New York: M. Evans and Company, Inc., 1982), p. 141.
9. Ibid.
10. Like the Student Recreation Center track, Bowling Green State University, Bowling Green, Ohio.
11. Like the Eppler South Complex track, Bowling Green State University, Bowling Green, Ohio.
12. Cooper, *The Aerobics Program for Total Well-Being*, p. 141.
13. Lenore R. Zohman, M.D., et al, *The Cardiologists' Guide to Fitness and Health Through Exercise*. (New York: Simon and Schuster, 1979), p. 87.
14. Cooper, Movie, "Run Dick, Run Jane."
15. Ibid.
16. Kenneth H. Cooper, *The Aerobics Way*. (New York: M. Evans and Company, Inc., 1977), p. 10.
17. National Vital Statistics Division, National Center for Health Statistics, Rockville, MD, 1984.
18. Americal College of Obstetricians and Gynecologists: *Safety Guidelines for Women Who Exercise*, No. 1, p. 6.
19. Zohman, p. 72.
20. *The Harvard Medical School Health Letter*, Volume X, No. 6, April 1985, p. 3.
21. Ibid.
22. Ibid.

Chapter 2

1. American College of Obstetricians and Gynecologists: *Safety Guidelines for Women Who Exercise* (ACOG Home Exercise Programs). Washington, D.C.: ACOG, 1986, p. 3.
2. Unpublished research date of Karen S. Mazzeo collected on students enrolled in aerobic dance courses, 1980-1986.
3. The American College of Sports Medicine, *Encyclopedia of Sport Sciences and Medicine* (New York: The Macmillan Company, 1971), p. 216.
4. Lenore Zohman, M.D., et al, *The Cardiologists' Guide to Fitness and Health Through Exercise* (New York: Simon and Schuster, 1979), p. 81.
5. ACOG, No. 11, p. 6
6. Unpublished research data of Karen S. Mazzeo collected on students enrolled in aerobic dance courses, 1984-1986.
7. ACOG, No. 5, p. 6.
8. Unpublished research data of Karren S. Mazzeo collected on students enrolled in aerobic dance courses, Spring 1986.
9. ACOG, No. 2, p. 6.
10. Ibid., p. 5.
11. Ibid.
12. Ibid.
13. Ibid., pp. 4-5.
14. Zohman, p. 87.

15. Michael Newton, M.D., Professor of Obstetrics and Gynecology at Northwestern Medical School and Director of Gynecologic Oncology at Prentice Women's Hospital and Maternity Center in Chicago, quoted viewpoints, June 1982.
16. Mazzeo, Spring 1986.
17. Ibid.
18. *The Harvard Medical School Health Letter,* Volume VIII, No. 10, August 1983, p. 2.

Chapter 4

1. Donald K. Mathews and Edward L. Fox, *The Physiological Basis of Physical Education and Athletics.* (Philadelphia: W.B. Saunders Company, 1976).
2. Bob Anderson, *Stretching.* (Bolinas, Calif.: Shelter Publications, 1980), pp. 9, 13.
3. Ibid., p. 13.
4. Carolyn O. Bowers, et al, *Judging and Coaching Women's Gymnastics.* (Palo Alto, Calif.: Mayfield Publishing Company, 1981), p. 336.
5. Ibid.

Chapter 6

1. American College of Obstetricians and Gynecologists: *Safety Guidelines for Women Who Exercise* (ACOG Home Exercise Programs). Washington, D.C., ACOG, 1986, p. 6.
2. John Patrick O'Shea, *Scientific Principles and Methods of Strength Fitness,* Second Edition. (Addison-Wesley Publishing Company: Reading, Mass., 1976), p. 89.
3. Bud Getchell, *Physical Fitness A Way of Life.* (New York: John Wiley and Sons, 1983), pp. 45-46.
4. Judy Alter, *Surviving Exercise.* (Boston: Houghton Mifflin Company, 1983), p. 38.

Chapter 7

1. *Collier's Encyclopedia 1981 Yearbook* (New York: Macmillan Educational Corporation, 1980), pp. 159,333.
2. Unpublished research data collected on students of aerobic dance in the Bowling Green (Ohio) University and community area, 1980-1986.
3. Ibid.
4. Ibid.
5. Norman Vincent Peale, *Positive Imaging.* (Pawling, N.Y.: Foundation for Christian Living, 1982), p. 94.
6. Anne Morrow Lindbergh, *Gift from the Sea.* (New York: Vintage Books, 1978), p. 56.
7. Roman G. Carek, Ph.D., Director of the Counseling and Career Development Center, Bowling Green State University, Bowling Green, Ohio, from his Stress Management presentation in the LIFE Seminar Workshop Series, 1982, held at the Student Recreation Center of BGSU.
8. Quoted remarks from psychologist and mental health educator, Dr. Murray Banks during a lecture series on mental hygiene, 1977.

Chapter 8

1. American College of Obstetricians and Gynecologists: *Safety Guidelines for Women Who Exercise* (ACOG Home Exercise Programs). Washington, D.C., ACOG, 1986, p. 6.

Chapter 9

1. Unpublished research data of Karen S. Mazzeo, collected on students enrolled in physical education general courses at Bowling Green State University, Bowling Green, Ohio, and the Bowling Green community area, 1980-1986.

2. W. Sheldon, *Atlas of Men*. (New York: Harper and Brothers, 1954), p. 120.
3. Pamphlet-brochure accompanying the RJL BIA-103 Body Composition Analyzer, RJL Systems, 9930 Whittier, Detroit, MI 48224.
4. Handout of Dr. Richard Bowers, Director, Sportsphysiology Laboratory, Bowling Green State University, Bowling Green, Ohio, 1978.
5. Jack H. Wilmore, Ph.D., "Anthropometric Estimate of Body Composition," paper delivered in the Fitness Section of 1972 AAHPER Convention, Houston, Texas.
6. Donald K. Mathews and Edward L. Fox, *The Physiological Basis of Physical Education and Athletics*. (Philadelphia: W.B. Saunders Company, 1976), p. 422.
7. Ibid., p. 423.
8. Pamphlet-brochure accompanying the RJL BIA-103 Body Composition Analyzer.
9. Ibid.
10. Jan Lewis, "Nutrition Notes. Dietary Guidelines 2," Bowling Green State University, Bowling Green, Ohio, 1981.
11. Richard Eppstein, Director, Better Business Bureau, Toledo, Ohio, during a lecture to Karen S. Mazzeo's class, January 1980.
12. William Gottlieb, "A Lifetime of Fitness" (views of Thomas Cureton, Ph.D.), *Prevention*, December 1, 1980, p. 54.
13. Lewis, "Nutrition Notes 2," p. 6.
14. Ibid., p. 4.
15. Ibid.
16. Ibid.
17. Thomas Gordon, Ph.D., P.E.T. *Parent Effectiveness Training*. (New York: Peter H. Wyden, Inc., 1970).

Chapter 10

1. National Dairy Council, "Guide to Wise Food Choices" B 170-1 (Rosemont, IL: National Dairy Council, 1978), p. 4.
2. National Dairy Council, "Guide to Good Eating . . . A Recommended Daily Pattern" B 164-5 (Rosemont, IL: National Dairy Council, 1980), 4th Edition, 1977.
3. Ibid.
4. National Dairy Council, "Guide to Wise Food Choices," p. 1.
5. Ibid., p. 4.
6. Ibid.
7. Ibid.
8. U.S. Department of Agriculture, U.S. Department of Health and Human Services, Home and Garden Bulletin No. 232, "Nutrition and Your Health, Dietary Guidelines for Americans," February 1980.
9. Jan Lewis, "Nutrition Notes: Nutrition and the Athlete" Workshop Series, Nutrition Education and Training Program, Bowling Green State University, Bowling Green, Ohio, 1981.
10. Ibid.
11. Nathan Smith, M.D., et al, *Handbook for the Young Athlete*. (Palo Alto, Calif.: Bull Publishing Co., 1978), p. 77.
12. Unpublished research data of Karen S. Mazzeo, collected on students of aerobic dance, 1980-1986.
13. *The Harvard Medical School Health Letter,* Volume II, No. 4, February 1986, p. 7.
14. Ibid., Volume X, No. 8, June 1985, p. 3.
15. Ibid., Volume II, No. 4, February 1986, p. 5.
16. Ibid., Volume X, No. 5, March 1985, p. 7.
17. Ibid., No. 8, June 1985, p. 6.
18. National Dairy Council, "Comprehensive List of Foods" B 082-5 (Rosemont, IL: National Dairy Council, 1978), pp. ii-viii.
19. Janet Lewis, Nutrition Education and Training Program, Director, Bowling Green State University, Bowling Green, Ohio, 1981—from handout developed. Sources are: Burger Chef Systems, Inc., Indianapolis, IN, 1978 (analyses obtained from USDA Handbook No. 8); Chart House, Inc., Oak Brook, IL, 1978; Nutrition analysis of food served at McDonald's Restaurants, WARF Institute, Inc., Madison, WI, June 1977; International Dairy Queen, Inc., Minneapolis, MN, 1978; Nutrition Content of Average Serving, Heublein Food Service and

Franchising Group, June 1976; Long John Silver's Seafood Shoppes, Jan. 8, 1978 (nutritional analysis information furnished in study conducted by the Department of Nutrition and Food Science, University of Kentucky); Research 900 and Pizza Hut, Inc., Wichita, KS; Menu Item Portions, July 1976, Taco Bell Co., San Antonio, TX., Adams CF: *Nutritive Value of American Foods in Common Units*, USDA Agricultural Research Service, Agriculture Handbook No. 456, November 1975; Church CF, Church HN: *Food Values of Portions Commonly Used*, ed. 12, Philadelphia, J.B. Lippincott Co., 1975; Valley Baptist Medical Center, Food Service Department: Descriptions of Mexican-American Foods, NASCO, Atkinson, WI; Adams CF: *Nutritive Value of American Foods in Common Units*, USDA Agricultural Research Service, Agriculture Handbook No. 456, November 1975; Coca-Cola Company, Atlanta, GA, January 1977; *American Hospital Formulatory Service*, Washington, American Society of Hospital Pharmacists, Section 28: 20, March 1978.

Chapter 11

1. Kenneth H. Cooper, M.D., M.P.H. *Running Without Fear*. (New York: M. Evans and Company, Inc.), 1985, p. 121.
2. Committee on Nutritional Misinformation, Food and Nutrition Board, National Research Council, National Academy of Sciences, "Water Deprivation and Performance of Athletics," distributed by the Nutrition Education and Training Program, Bowling Green State University, 1981.
3. The American College of Sports Medicine, *Encyclopedia of Sport Sciences and Medicine* (New York: The Macmillan Company, 1971), p. 215.
4. Ibid., p. 216.
5. *The Harvard Medical School Health Letter,* Volume VIII, No. 2, p. 4.
6. The American College of Sports Medicine, p. 216.
7. Interview with Jane Steinberg, Athletic Trainer of Intercollegiate Sports at Bowling Green State University, Bowling Green, Ohio, Spring 1982.
8. American College of Obstetricians and Gynecologists: *Safety Guidelines for Women Who Exercise* (ACOG Home Exercise Programs). Washington, D.C., ACOG, 1986, p. 6.
9. Interview, Steinberg, 1982.
10. Orthotic for sports shoe prescribed and dispensed by Dr. Charles Marlowe, Podiatrist to Karen S. Mazzeo, summer 1983, with accompanying brochure of information.
11. *The Harvard Medical School Health Letter,* Volume XI, No. 5, p. 4.
12. *Runner's World,* "Runner's World Reviews What's New in Running Bras," June 1986, p. 92.
13. Michael Newton, M.D., Professor of Obstetrics and Gynecology at Northwestern Medical School and Director of Gynecologic Oncology at Prentice Women's Hospital and Maternity Center in Chicagjo, quoted viewpoints, June 1982.
14. Ibid.
15. Ibid.
16. Ibid.
17. Michael Newton, M.D., and Edward R. Newton, M.D., *Complications in Gynecology and Obstetrics: Operations, Procedures, and Treatments.* (Philadelphia: W.B. Saunders Company; in press 1986), manuscript, p. 74 of Chapter 10.
18. Ibid.
19. Newton, quoted viewpoints, June 1982.
20. Cooper, *Running Without Fear,* p. 128.

Appendix

CHART 1
A Commitment Contract is Made

I (name) _____ am

determined that today (date) _____ I am

committed to becoming fit!

I acknowledge that I am in need of improvement in various facets of my well-being (physical, social, emotional,

intellectual) and commit to devote _____ minutes **EVERY** day toward making positive change in my

fitness habits. This is in addition to the time spent in class.

The best time for me to work on this change is _____ AM/PM.

Absolutely **NOTHING** will take presidence over this block of time that I have set aside to experience personal

fitness gains.

Signed _____

This commitment was witnessed by* _____

*By witnessing this, make it your responsibility to *positively encourage* the individual toward reaching the goal(s) he/she sets.

CHART 2
Index Card of Information –
A Profile on You

In order to maintain a profile on students who enroll in a class, it is important to keep a few statistics so that change can be noted and statistics developed for future reference. Please fill in the following information, remove carefully from the textbook, and give to your instructor.

NAME _____ RANK:F/So/J/S/Grad/Other

ADDRESS ON CAMPUS _____ PHONE_____

AGE _____ HEIGHT _____ WEIGHT _____ SKINFOLD _____ IDEAL WEIGHT_____

RATE YOUR FITNESS LEVEL: SUPERIOR/EXCELLENT/GOOD/FAIR/POOR/VERY POOR-PRE
                          SUPERIOR/EXCELLENT/GOOD/FAIR/POOR/VERY POOR-POST

PREVIOUS CLASS OR INSTRUCTION IN COURSE:_____

SPORTS IN WHICH YOU PARTICIPATE/ENJOY ON A WEEKLY BASIS:_____

REASON(S) FOR TAKING COURSE:_____

DID ANYONE RECOMMEND THIS COURSE OR INSTRUCTOR? _____

PHYSICAL LIMITATIONS _____

FOLD OUT HERE

ACTIVITY THAT YOU WOULD LIKE FOR ME TO BE SURE TO COVER:_____

HEART RATE.   RESTING _____ TRANING ZONE _____

DO YOU TAKE *ANY* DRUG TO ALTER YOUR HEART RATE ?_____

DO YOU DESIRE TO: (CIRCLE) GAIN LEAN WEIGHT/LOSE FAT WEIGHT/STAY SAME

DO YOU SMOKE? _____ IF SO, NUMBER PER DAY?_____

RATE YOUR ALCOHOL CONSUMPTION: NEVER/DAILY/ _____

DO YOU CHEW: GUM/TOBACCO/OBJECTS/FINGERNAILS

LIST INTEREST IN MUSIC, FAVORITE SONG, FAVORITE ARTIST:_____

OTHER INTERESTS _____

IF 35 OR OLDER, OR HAVE SPECIFIC LIMITATIONS: I HAVE MY DOCTOR'S PERMISSION TO PARTICIPATE

_____

DOCTOR'S NAME AND PHONE: _____

I have read and understand the responsibilities for participants and the instructor.

_____   _____
                    Signature   **Date**

CHART 3
Profile of Information Index
For Laboratory Stress Testing

Symptoms

Family history

Blood pressure

Total cholesterol/HDL ratio

Blood sugar

Resting ECG

Other:

Results & Recommendations

CHART 4
Pre Physical Fitness Testing
and Appraisal Results

Name: _____ Age: _____ Sex: _____

PRE-TEST:

Cooper's Twelve-Minute and 1.5-Mile Test

Appraisal was (circle): Before / During / After   Aerobics Program

A. Cooper Twelve-Minute Run/Walk Test

  Start Time: _____ Stop Time: _____ Distance Covered: _____

  Check Table 1-1 for Fitness Category.

B. 12 minute run/walk test on a 190 yd. track:

  Start Time: _____ Stop Time: _____

  Check Off Laps: 1 - 2 - 3 - 4 - 5 - 6 - 7 - 8 - 9 - 10 - 11 - 12 - 13 - 14 - 15 - 16 - 17 - 18

  Check Table 1-2 for Fitness Category.

C. 12 minute run/walk test on a 126 yd. track:

  Start Time: _____ Stop Time: _____

  Check Off Laps: 1 - 2 - 3 - 4 - 5 - 6 - 7 - 8 - 9 - 10 - 11 - 12 - 13 - 14 - 15 - 16 - 17 - 18 - 19 - 20 - 21 - **22 - 23 - 24 - 25 - 26 - 27**

  Check Table 1-3 for Fitness Category.

D. **Cooper 1.5 Mile Run/Walk Test:**

  Check Off Laps: (14 for 190 yd. track; 21 for 126 yd. track):

  1 - 2 - 3 - 4 - 5 - 6 - 7 - 8 - 9 - 10 - 11 - 12 - 13 - 14 - 15 - 16 - 17 - 18 - 19 - 20 - 21

  Or:

  Stop Time: _____

  − Start Time: _____   Just record here if
                                              using an open roadway.

  Time: _____

  Check Table 1-4 for Fitness Category.

Circle Fitness Category: Very Poor / Poor / Fair / Good / Excellent / Superior

-Over-

CHART 5
Post Physical Fitness Testing and Appraisal Results

Name: _____ Age: _____ Sex: _____

POST-TEST:

Cooper's Twelve-Minute and 1.5-Mile Test

Appraisal was (circle): Before / During / After   Aerobics Program
A. Cooper Twelve-Minute Run/Walk Test
   Start Time: _____ Stop Time: _____ Distance Covered: _____
   Check Table 1-1 for Fitness Category.

B. 12 minute run/walk test on a 190 yd. track:
   Start Time: _____ Stop Time: _____
    Check Off Laps: 1 - 2 - 3 - 4 - 5 - 6 - 7 - 8 - 9 - 10 - 11 - 12 - 13 - 14 - 15 - 16 - 17 - 18
   Check Table 1-2 for Fitness Category.

C. 12 minute run/walk test on a 126 yd. track:
   Start Time: _____ Stop Time: _____
   Check Off Laps: 1 - 2 - 3 - 4 - 5 - 6 - 7 - 8 - 9 - 10 - 11 - 12 - 13 - 14 - 15 - 16 - 17 - 18 - 19 - 20 - 21 - 22 - 23 - 24 - 25 - 26 - 27
   Check Table 1-3 for Fitness Category.

D. Cooper 1.5 Mile Run/Walk Test
   Check Off Laps: (14 for 190 yd. track; 21 for 126 yd. track):
   1 - 2 - 3 - 4 - 5 - 6 - 7 - 8 - 9 - 10 - 11 - 12 - 13 - 14 - 15 - 16 - 17 - 18 - 19 - 20 - 21

Or:

Stop Time: _____

− Start Time: _____   Just record here if
                                using an open roadway.

Time: _____
   Check Table 1-4 for Fitness Category.

Circle Fitness Category: Very Poor / Poor / Fair / Good / Excellent / Superior

CHART 6
Plotting Your Resting Heart Rate

Establishing RsHR

WEEK I:

Day 1:_____

Day 2:_____

Day 3:_____

Day 4:_____

Day 5:_____

Sum Total:_____

÷5: _____ RsHR

Week		II		III		IV		V		VI		VII		VIII		IX		X	
Class	1	2	1	2	1	2	1	2	1	2	1	2	1	2	1	2	1	2
Bi-Weekly Resting Heart Rate																		
120																		
115																		
110																		
105																		
100																		
95																		
90																		
85																		
80																		
75																		
70																		
65																		
60																		
55																		
50																		
45																		
40																		
35																		
30																		

NOTE: Take your resting heart rate at the first possibility in the A.M., before arising. Use first two fingers at thumb side of wrist, carotid artery in neck, temple area, or other pulse point.

Resting H.R.—Week I: _____   At Finish: _____   (-)Loss/(+)Gain: _____

CHART 7

How to Figure Your Training Zone

Since three basic factors enter into figuring your estimated safe exercise zone, those must be established first:

1.   Your current **age:**_____

2.   How **active** is your **life-style?** _____ _____ **% MHR. If you are:**
     • Sedentary: use the figure **60-69%** of your maximum heart rate (but **only** for the first two or three **weeks**)
     • Moderately physically active: use **70-75%** of your maximum heart rate.

3.   Your average **resting heart rate** (established on Chart 6): _____

Now place your numbers in the formula that follows:

A. 220   -_____ = _____ **Estimated Maximal Heart Rate (MHR)**
          (Index number)   (Your Age)

B. _____ -_____ = _____
          MHR   Resting HR   HR Reserve

C. _____ × •_____ = _____ + **Resting H.R.** = _____ *
     Heart Rate Reserve   Lower end life-style activity range
                              (i.e. #2 above)

     _____ × •_____ = _____ + **Resting H.R.** = _____ *
     Heart Rate Reserve   Higher end life-style activity range
                              (i.e. #2 above)

RANGE OF   _____ * This range is your **estimated safe exercise zone.** Keep your heart rate
YOUR   working in this range while you aerobically exercise for 20-30 minutes of
TARGET   _____ * each session.

                              Re-figure as you "age," as you can reclassify your "lifestyle" of activity, or
                              as you have a marked decline in your resting heart rate.

For example: Chris is 20 years old, a moderately active person (70-75% range), with a resting heart rate of 62.

A. 220 - 20 = 200 MHR

B. 200 - 62 = 138 Heart Rate Reserve

C. 138 × .70 = 96 + 62 =158*   Training Zone Heart Rate
     138 × .75 = 104 + 62 =166*

If Chris keeps working (aerobic dancing) the range of 158 to 166 heartbeats per minute the heart would be **safely** working toward the training effect.

CHART 8
Aerobics Heart Rate Monitoring

Name: _____ Date: _____ Class: _____

Training Zone: _____ — _____ Initial Resting H.R. Average_____

Directions: Check heart rate **immediately after** for 6 seconds. Add a zero and record as **"I" reading**(Immediate). Keep walking. After **one minute,** check heart rate again for 15 seconds. Multiply by 4 and record, as **"R" reading** (Recovery). First two weeks will also include immediate readings which do not reflect the training zone (i.e., Before Activity H.R. and After Warmup).

WEEK 1		**WEEK 2**		**WEEK 3**	
CLASS 1 (At Home)	Class 2	CLASS 1 (At Home)	CLASS 2	CLASS 1 (At Home)	CLASS 2
Resting H.R.: 1 ____/2 ____/3 ____/4 ____/5 ____		Resting H.R.:_____ _____		Resting H.R.:_____ _____	
Before Activity H.R. _____ _____		_____ _____		_____ _____	
After Stretching Warmup _____ _____		_____ _____		Aerobic Intervals	
Comments	Aerobic Interval Readings			I / R	I / R
	I / R	I / R	I / R	I: ___ / ___	___ / ___
				II: ___ / ___	___ / ___
Jog/Jump Rope	I. ____ / ____	___ / ___	___ / ___	III: ___ / ___	___ / ___
Dance	II. ____ / ____	___ / ___	___ / ___	IV: ___ / ___	___ / ___
Dance	III. ____ / ____	___ / ___	___ / ___	V: ___ / ___	___ / ___
				VI: ___ / ___	___ / ___
After Cool Down_____ _____				After Conscious Relaxation	After Conscious Relaxation
	Below 120?	Below 120?	Below 120?	_____ _____	
After Strength Training_____ _____				Below 120?	Below 120?
				_____ _____	
Comments:	Comments:	Comments:	Comments:	Comments:	Comments:

(At Home)	**WEEK 4**		**WEEK 5**		**WEEK 6**		**WEEK 7**	
	CLASS 1	**CLASS 2**	**CLASS 1**	**CLASS 2**	**CLASS 1**	**CLASS 2**	**CLASS 1**	**CLASS 2**
Resting H.R.	_____	_____	_____	_____	_____	_____	_____	_____
Before Activity H.R.	_____	_____	_____	_____	_____	_____	_____	_____
Aerobic Intervals	I / R	I / R	I / R	I / R	I / R	I / R	I / R	I / R
I:	__/__	__/__	__/__	__/__	__/__	__/__	__/__	__/__
II:	__/__	__/__	__/__	__/__	__/__	__/__	__/__	__/__
III:	__/__	__/__	__/__	__/__	__/__	__/__	__/__	__/__
IV:	__/__	__/__	__/__	__/__	__/__	__/__	__/__	__/__
V:	__/__	__/__	__/__	__/__	__/__	__/__	__/__	__/__
VI:	__/__	__/__	__/__	__/__	__/__	__/__	__/__	__/__
VII:	__/__	__/__	__/__	__/__	__/__	__/__	__/__	__/__
VIII:	__/__	__/__	__/__	__/__	__/__	__/__	__/__	__/__
IX:	__/__	__/__	__/__	__/__	__/__	__/__	__/__	__/__
X:	__/__	__/__	__/__	__/__	__/__	__/__	__/__	__/__
	After Conscious Relaxation		After Conscious Relaxation		After Conscious Relaxation		After Conscious Relaxation	
	Below 120 Comments	Below 120? Comments	Below 120? Comments	Below 120? Comments	Below 120? Comments	Below 120? Comments	Below 120? Comments	Below 120? Comments

(At Home)	**WEEK 8**		**WEEK 9**		**WEEK 10**		List personal observations made on all heart rate monitoring, noting any dramatic changes:
	Class 1	Class 2	Class 1	Class 2	Class 1	Class 2	
Resting HR:	_____	_____	_____	_____	_____	_____	
Before Activity HR:	_____	_____	_____	_____	_____	_____	
Aerobic Intervals	I / R	I / R	I / R	I / R	I / R	I / R	
I:	__/__	__/__	__/__	__/__	__/__	__/__	
II:	__/__	__/__	__/__	__/__	__/__	__/__	
III:	__/__	__/__	__/__	__/__	__/__	__/__	
IV:	__/__	__/__	__/__	__/__	__/__	__/__	
V:	__/__	__/__	__/__	__/__	__/__	__/__	
VI:	__/__	__/__	__/__	__/__	__/__	__/__	
VII:	__/__	__/__	__/__	__/__	__/__	__/__	
VIII:	__/__	__/__	__/__	__/__	__/__	__/__	
IX:	__/__	__/__	__/__	__/__	__/__	__/__	
X:	__/__	__/__	__/__	__/__	__/__	__/__	
	After Conscious Relaxation		After Conscious Relaxation		After Conscious Relaxation		
	Below 120? Comments	Below 120? Comments	Below 120? Comments	Below 120? Comments	Below 120? Comments	Below 120? Comments	

CHART 9
Reflecting Upon Your Emotions

I: Frequently Used Stress Releases:	II. Stressors Which Trigger Your Need To React This Way:	III. Rate your Usage:			
		A	F	O	N
Alcohol usage	_____	_____			
Become very quiet	_____	_____			
Chew gum	_____	_____			
Chew your nails	_____	_____			
Chew objects (pencils/toothpicks)	_____	_____			
Cry	_____	_____			
Drink coffee-tea-cola	_____	_____			
Draw artistically	_____	_____			
Drug usage	_____	_____			
Eat without monitoring	_____	_____			
Exercise strenuously	_____	_____			
Get lost in a good book	_____	_____			
Go off somewhere to be alone	_____	_____			
Hit people; kick animals	_____	_____			
Laugh hysterically	_____	_____			
Play a musical instrument	_____	_____			
Play loud stereo music	_____	_____			
Profanity	_____	_____			
Religious resort to prayer/reading	_____	_____			
Sex discriminately/indiscriminately	_____	_____			
Sleep	_____	_____			
Smoke cigarettes	_____	_____			
Take over-the-counter drugs (aspirin/antacids)	_____	_____			
Talk on phone	_____	_____			
Tease	_____	_____			
Throw objects	_____	_____			
Write feelings on paper (letters; diary)	_____	_____			
Work with your hands (creatively making things)	_____	_____			
Yell and scream	_____	_____			

Others: _____

Directions:

I. Read this column slowly & mentally identify if you use this release.

II. Write what stressor would set you off to use this release.

III. How often? **A**lways; **F**requently; **O**ccasionally; **N**ever.

IV. Possible Stressful Situations:

Select a response from Column I on the other side & write in the blank.

Someone telling you that you need to lose (or gain) weight_____

Studying 5 hours consecutively_____

First awaken in the morning_____

Antics of children or babies_____

Unreasonable roommate activity_____

Watching four TV "soaps" in a row_____

See an advertisement for a "binge" food_____

Parental pressure (grades, money)_____

Fail exam in course_____

Watching an exciting sports event in person_____

After a tedious 8-hour work day_____

Receiving a huge parking fine_____

Long lines_____

Before a speech_____

Waiting for a long overdue (*late*) friend_____

Budgeting your bills_____

Cleanliness of room/roommate_____

Messiness of room/roommate_____

Hearing unjust gossip about yourself_____

After a heated argument_____

Criticism of your efforts_____

In the company of strangers_____

Must do before you go to sleep_____

Note Star (*) those negative stress releases you use & wish to improve upon or totally change.

V. What I've learned about myself and my positive and negative reactions to stressful situations:

VI. One Resolution or goal:

CHART 10
Choreographing Your Own Routines

Aerobic Dance Choreographed Routines

Easy **Choreography:**

** Wide stride w̄ arms cross-over	2X
* Jog	32X
* Polka	16X
* Doubles: knees & kicks	4X
* Hustle w̄ knee-lift & clap	8X
* Rock F/B	8X
* Rock side/side	8X
* Hopscotch	8X
* Charleston	2X

_____

*Repeat all 3X (omit **)

*Jog to end

Suggested Song: "*Holding Out for a Hero*" from *Footloose,* Bonnie Tyler.

Moderate Difficulty

* A-B-C-D Pattern (4's) & reversed ea.
  16 cts: 2X
* Jog F/B 8X each
* Jazz touch 4X S/S; 4X F/B (8X total)
* Step-hop-step-kick: 6X
* Rock F/B: 8X
* Jump 'n clap, circling 8 cts: 2X
* Side stride-jumps 'n claps: 8X
* Arm sweeps up (standing wide stride)
  8 cts: 1X
* Arm sweeps down (standing wide stride)
  8 cts: 1X
* Knee-lift elbow touch 8 cts: 2X
* Knee-lift elbow touch-crossed 8 cts: 2X

_____

* Repeat all, 3X

Suggested Song: "*Jump For My Love*" by Pointer Sisters.

Now You Choreograph:

List 8 favorite basic step/gesture patterns:
Give repetitions:

Patterns	Reps.	Total Cts.
* Introduction move: _____	_____ X =	_____CTS.
* _____	_____ X =	_____CTS.
* _____	_____ X =	_____CTS.
* _____	_____ X =	_____CTS.
* _____	_____ X =	_____CTS.
* _____	_____ X =	_____CTS.
* _____	_____ X =	_____CTS.
* _____	_____ X =	_____CTS.

_____

* Repeat all _____ Times.
* Conclusion to end move: _____ = _____CTS.

List 10 coordination patterns & basics:
Give repetitions:

* Introductory move: _____	_____ X =	_____CTS.
* _____	_____ X =	_____CTS.
* _____	_____ X =	_____CTS.
* _____	_____ X =	_____CTS.
* _____	_____ X =	_____CTS.
* _____	_____ X =	_____CTS.
* _____	_____ X =	_____CTS.
* _____	_____ X =	_____CTS.
* _____	_____ X =	_____CTS.
* _____	_____ X =	_____CTS.

_____

* Repeat all _____ Times.
* Conclusion to end move: _____ = _____CTS.

CHART 10
Advanced Choreography To Specific Song:

	First Time:	Repeats:	
		1st	2nd
"*Fame*," Irene Cara			
I. Jog Beg. & End	16X	-	-
II. Side - Together - Side - Touch Pattern	4X		
Side - Touch - Side - Kick	2X	X	X
Quad 'n Ham Pattern	2X		

III.	Slide - S - S - Jump Clap Knee-Lift Hop & Slap, Circling 8 Cts.	4X 2X	-	XX
IV.	Fwd. 3 Jogs; Hold; Push-Pull Arms (4 Cts.) Bk. 3 Jogs; Hold; Push-Pull Arms (4 Cts.) Cha-Cha & Kick Pattern	8 Cts. 8 Cts. 2X	X	-
V.	Stride 'n Twist Pattern	4X	X	-
VI.	"Fame" - Widestride Arms & Legs Jump & Hold Fwd. Jog 8X, Bk. Jog 8X, Repeat Side Jazz Touch F/B Jazz Touch Hip Thrust 'N Click	4 Cts. 32 Cts. 4X 3X 8X	X	XX

ADVANCED Choreography To Specific Song:

Song: "New Attitude," By Patti LaBelle, MCA Records

Sequence	Activity > You Choreograph	8 Counts	Total Counts	Lyrics
I.		2	16	Instrumental
II.		4	32	Added Instrumental
		4	32	Added Instrumental
III.		4	32	. . . Running
		4	32	I took it
IV.	(Chorus)	2	16	Somehow
		4	32	I'm feeling
		4	32	I'm in control
V.		I	8	Instrumental
	Repeats	III - IV (Chorus) - V III - IV (Chorus)	-	296	. . . I'm wearing . . . O-O-O!
VI.		4	32 ⌉	Feeling blue
		4	32	96
		4	32 ⌋	

CHART 11
Your Current Body Composition and Ideal Weight

Directions: Figure out your specific data by using the formula below.

• Your current nude weight, in pounds: _____

• Your current skinfold measurement, in millimeters: _____

Wilmore's* formula for the anthropometric estimate of body composition:

STEP 1 LBW (lean body weight):

Women:

20.20

+ _____._____ = (.635 x your weight in pounds)

_____._____ = a subtotal of above

− _____._____ = (.503 x your subscapular skinfold, in mm.)

_____._____ = LBW

Men:

22.62

+ _____._____ = (.793 x your weight in pounds)

_____._____ = a subtotal of above

− _____._____ = (.801 x your abdominal skinfold, in mm.)

_____._____ = LBW

STEP 2 % FAT:

$$\frac{\text{Body Weight-LBW}}{\text{Body Weight}} \times 100 = \underline{\hspace{2cm}} \text{ Current \% Fat}$$

*Wilmore, Jack H., Ph.D., University of Texas, Austin.

Categories:

	Women		Men
	30%	Obesity	20%
	25%	Overweight	15%
	22-20%	Ideal	12½-10%
	Below 20%	Underfat	Below 10%

Thus, I am currently in which category? _____

_____

STEP 3 RELATIVE WEIGHTS FOR YOU:

Women:			Men:
$\frac{\text{LBW}}{.70}$ = _____	Your "Obesity" Weight _____	=	$\frac{\text{LBW}}{.80}$
$\frac{\text{LBW}}{.75}$ = _____	Your "Overweight" Weight _____	=	$\frac{\text{LBW}}{.85}$
$\frac{\text{LBW}}{.78}$ = _____	Your "High Ideal" Weight _____	=	$\frac{\text{LBW}}{.875}$
$\frac{\text{LBW}}{.80}$ = _____	Your "Low Ideal" Weight _____	=	$\frac{\text{LBW}}{.90}$
Below The Above Figure = _____	Your "Underfat" Weight _____	=	Below The Above Figure

Thus, when you step on a scale and weigh the above weight(s) **at your current lean weight,** you can classify yourself into one of the four previously listed categories: obesity, overweight, high to low ideal weight range, or underfat range. The ideal precentage of fat to lean weight—called your "ideal weight"—is a **three-pound range,** not just one figure.

CHART 12

Recording Weight Maintenance, Loss, and/or Gain

(*Due this week of class)

Weeks		I	II	III	IV	V	VI	VII	VIII	IX	X*
Pounds	15										
	14										
	13										
	12										
	11										
	10										
	9										
	8										
	7										
	6										
	5										
	4										
	3										
	2										
Gain (lbs.)	1										
Starting Wt.	0										
Loss (lbs,)	1										
	2										
	3										
	4										
	5										
	6										
	7										
	8										
	9										
	10										
	11										
	12										
	13										
	14										
	15										
	16										
	17										
	18										
	19										
	20										

NOTE: Weigh yourself once a week, first possibility in AM, after elimination and before first meal.

Start of class weight: _____ End of class weight: _____ +/− Total: _____

NOTE: It is physiologically impossible to lose more than approximately 2 pounds of FAT per week.

Directions:
1) Record your starting weight at zero area and where it states "starting weight," and under graph "start of class weight.
2) Weigh once a week, first thing in the morning *after* arising, *after* elimination, and *before* you eat breakfast. This is the most accurate time of the day to weigh.
3) Record a maintenance weight in zero block line, or directly *next to* your last recorded weight.
4) Record weight *gain* pounds as plus numbers of blocks *up* from the last recorded weight.
5) Record weight *loss* pounds *down* from the last recorded weight.
6) Record a final weight where it states "ending weight."
7) Determine a final *total* maintenance gain or loss figure where it states "+/− _____ weight for 10 week period."

CHART 13

My Daily Consumption

WEEK 1:

	DATE/ TODAY	/	/	/	/	/	/	/
MILK 1 2								
MEAT 1 2								
FRUIT & VEG. 1 2 3 4								
GRAIN 1 2 3 4								
TOTAL Calories From Above:	1200	1200	1200	1200	1200	1200	1200	
Other (i.e. "junk food") Calories:								
Extra (servings) Calories:								
TOTAL DAILY CALORIC INTAKE:								

CHART 14

My Daily Consumption—continued

WEEK 2:

	DATE/ TODAY						
MILK 1 2							
MEAT 1 2							
FRUIT & VEG. 1 2 3 4							
GRAIN 1 2 3 4							
TOTAL Calories From Above:	1200	1200	1200	1200	1200	1200	1200
Other (i.e. "junk food") Calories:							
Extra (servings) Calories:							
TOTAL DAILY CALORIC INTAKE:							

(a) What groups do you eat with consistent regularity? _____

(b) Which groups do you tend to slight? _____

(c) In which groups and categories do you tend to overeat? _____

CHART 15

Approximate Energy Cost of Various Activities

I. My weight in lbs. _____

(One lb = .454 Kgs.) <u>x .454</u>

My Kg. wt. is: _____ *Place this number under column II.

Activity	Calories per minute per kilograms of body weight	II. Multiply Times Your Kg. Wt.*		III. Calories Burned/ Min.	Record the Duration of Mins. Spent Here		IV. Energy Expended Per Activity Today
1. Sleep	.0171	×	=	_____	×	_____	=	_____
2. Rest in bed	.0172	×	=	_____	×	_____	=	_____
3. Lie at ease	.0174	×	=	_____	×	_____	=	_____
4. Sit at ease	.0176	×	=	_____	×	_____	=	_____
5. Read	.0176	×	=	_____	×	_____	=	_____
6. Eat	.0204	×	=	_____	×	_____	=	_____
7. Typing	.0209	×	=	_____	×	_____	=	_____
8. Writing	.0266	×	=	_____	×	_____	=	_____
9. Sit talking	.0269	×	=	_____	×	_____	=	_____
10. Play cards	.0209	×	=	_____	×	_____	=	_____
11. Pray or meditate	.0199	×	=	_____	×	_____	=	_____
12. Stand at ease	.0206	×	=	_____	×	_____	=	_____
13. Stand talking	.0308	×	=	_____	×	_____	=	_____
14. Stand light activity	.0352	×	=	_____	×	_____	=	_____
15. Toilet activities	.0276	×	=	_____	×	_____	=	_____
17. Washing	.0382	×	=	_____	×	_____	=	_____
18. Dressing	.0464	×	=	_____	×	_____	=	_____
19. Make bed	.0572	×	=	_____	×	_____	=	_____
22. DANCE EASY	**.053**	×	=	_____	×	_____	=	_____
23. DANCE MODERATELY	**.0971**	×	=	_____	×	_____	=	_____
24. DANCE HARD	**.1439**	×	=	_____	×	_____	=	_____
26. Racquetball light	.143	×	=	_____	×	_____	=	_____
27. Racquetball moderate	.179	×	=	_____	×	_____	=	_____
28. Racquetball hard	.215	×	=	_____	×	_____	=	_____
29. Bowling	.04	×	=	_____	×	_____	=	_____
30. Tennis doubles	.071	×	=	_____	×	_____	=	_____
31. Tennis moderate	.1	×	=	_____	×	_____	=	_____
32. Tennis hard	.157	×	=	_____	×	_____	=	_____
33. Soccer moderate	.1	×	=	_____	×	_____	=	_____
34. Soccer hard	.215	×	=	_____	×	_____	=	_____
35. Basketball moderate	.145	×	=	_____	×	_____	=	_____
36. Basketball hard	.215	×	=	_____	×	_____	=	_____
37. Golf with cart	.071	×	=	_____	×	_____	=	_____

Activity	Calories per minute per kilograms of body weight	II. Multiply Times Your Kg. Wt.*		III. Calories Burned/ Min.		Record the Duration of Mins. Spent Here		IV. Energy Expended Per Activity Today
38. Bike 6 mph	.063	×	=	_____	×	_____	=	_____
39. Bike 10 mph	.099	×	=	_____	×	_____	=	_____
40. Bike 13 mph	.155	×	=	_____	×	_____	=	_____
41. Bike 17 mph	.199	×	=	_____	×	_____	=	_____
42. Bike race	.223	×	=	_____	×	_____	=	_____
44. Walk 2 mph	.0357	×	=	_____	×	_____	=	_____
45. Walk 2.5 mph	.0429	×	=	_____	×	_____	=	_____
46. Walk 3 mph	.0529	×	=	_____	×	_____	=	_____
47. Walk 3.5 mph	.06	×	=	_____	×	_____	=	_____
48. Walk 4 mph	.0786	×	=	_____	×	_____	=	_____
49. Walk 4.5 mph	.1	×	=	_____	×	_____	=	_____
50. Walk 5 mph	.1186	×	=	_____	×	_____	=	_____
51. Walk 3 mph 10% grade	.1214	×	=	_____	×	_____	=	_____
53. Run 11 min/mi	.1442	×	=	_____	×	_____	=	_____
54. Run 10 min/mi	.1714	×	=	_____	×	_____	=	_____
55. Run 8.5 min/mi	.2	×	=	_____	×	_____	=	_____
56. Run 7.5 min/mi	.2229	×	=	_____	×	_____	=	_____
57. Run 6.7 min/mi	.25	×	=	_____	×	_____	=	_____
58. Run 6 min/mi	.28	×	=	_____	×	_____	=	_____
59. Run 5.5 min/mi	.31	×	=	_____	×	_____	=	_____
60. Run 5 min/mi	.35	×	=	_____	×	_____	=	_____
61. Swim Free 2 min/100	.156	×	=	_____	×	_____	=	_____
62. Swim Free 1.45 min/100	.194	×	=	_____	×	_____	=	_____
63. Swim Free 1.30 min/100	.24	×	=	_____	×	_____	=	_____
64. Swim Breast 2 min/100	.15	×	=	_____	×	_____	=	_____
65. Swim Back 2 min/100	.131	×	=	_____	×	_____	=	_____
66. Drive, automatic	.0384	×	=	_____	×	_____	=	_____
67. Drive, manual	.0398	×	=	_____	×	_____	=	_____
68. Drive, motorcycle	.0398	×	=	_____	×	_____	=	_____
69. Walk, downstairs	.0975	×	=	_____	×	_____	=	_____
70. Walk, upstairs	.254	×	=	_____	×	_____	=	_____

_____ = **V.**

VI. Total daily caloric intake is: _____ (see Chapter 9).

Total daily caloric expenditure is _____ (see above, V.)

Note: If these tables are the *same,* or quite close, you'll be at "weight maintenance" and you'll stay at the weight you're currently at. If intake is higher than expenditure, you'll probably *gain* weight. If intake is lower than expenditure, you'll probably *lose* weight.

Above activities and calories per minute per kilogram of body weight are from research, publications, and software developed by Dr. Frank M. Powell, Professor of Health, Physical Education, Furman University, Greenville, South Carolina 29613. It is available with complete directions as "Energy Expenditure Determination" software to be used on Apple IIe, @ $10.00.